Coping With Osteoarthritis

Robert H. Phillips, Ph.D.

AVERY PUBLISHING GROUP INC.
Garden City Park, New York

The medical information and procedures contained in this book are not intended as a substitute for consulting your physician. All matters regarding your physical health should be supervised by a medical professional.

Cover art by Tim Peterson
Cover design by Martin Hochberg and Rudy Shur
In-house editor Cynthia J. Eriksen
Typesetting by Multifacit Graphics, Keyport, NJ

Library of Congress Cataloging-in-Publication Data

Phillips, Robert H., 1948–
Coping with osteoarthritis : a guide to living with OA for you and your family / Robert H. Phillips.
p. cm.
Bibliography: p.
Includes index.
ISBN 0-89529-393-5 : $9.95
1. Osteoarthritis--Popular works. 2. Osteoarthritis--Psychological aspects. 3. Adjustment (Psychology) I. Title.
RC931.067P45 1989
616.7'22--dc19 89-175
CIP

Printed in the United States of America

10 9 8 7 6 5

Contents

Dedication

In order to cope most effectively, we benefit from the love and support of the people closest to us. I am therefore most grateful to the following special people, to whom this book is dedicated: to my wife, Sharon; my three sons, Michael, Larry, and Steven; my parents; my sister; my grandparents; all my other relatives and in-laws; and my friends.

Acknowledgements

I'd like to express appreciative words of thanks to some wonderful people who provided valuable assistance in the preparation of this book. Thanks to Robert Marcus, M.D., for his critical review, helpful suggestions and information, and enthusiastic participation in this project. Thanks to William Given, M.D., for his insightful review of the manuscript. Thanks to Sharon Balaban for the long hours that she spent painstakingly transcribing, revising, and typing the final manuscript. Finally, grateful thanks to Roland Moskowitz, M.D., for a professional evaluation of the highest caliber.

Foreword

Osteoarthritis, also known as degenerative joint disease, is the most common form of arthritis, affecting 20 million or more Americans. Many people (including, at times, physicians!) look at osteoarthritis as a "nuisance" that causes some mild aches and pains but never really incapacitates people. Unfortunately, in many individuals it is more than a minor problem, and can lead to significant pain, limitation, and overall disability, particularly when it involves significant joints such as the hips, knees, or spine. The enormity of the problem posed by osteoarthritis is seen in the statistics, which show that after age seventy, up to 85 percent of the general population has evidence of this disorder; in approximately 25 percent of these cases, the symptoms may be severe enough to require some form of treatment. Another common misconception is that little can be done to relieve osteoarthritis symptoms and that seeking help is without benefit. On the contrary, much can be done in the way of symptomatic relief; at times, joint protection may slow down the disease process.

Dr. Phillips has written an admirable book on how to cope with the disease. In order to cope successfully, you have to understand what the disorder is; this is outlined with clarity in sections describing what the disease is, how it is diagnosed, and how it is treated. Important questions, such as how pain can be handled, what effects special diets do (or do not) have, and when exercise or rest is appropriate, are all considered in balanced fashion. Other sections deal with how patients and families handle the disease, and how someone with OA can lead a healthy, wholesome existence while still not ignoring the important do's of management.

Chronic diseases are tough to handle—nobody teaches us how to do this while we're growing up! Dr. Phillips has put together a volume replete with understanding, sensitivity, and humor. He provides a common-sense approach to management and coping, which, if followed, will reduce the impact of this disorder on everyday life. What you can do, not what you can't do, is stressed. (Life has enough don'ts without adding to them unnecessarily!) The concepts can be carried over to other stresses in everyday life. I look forward to recommending this volume to my many patients with this disorder.

Roland W. Moskowitz, M.D.
Professor of Medicine
Case Western Reserve University
Director, Division of Rheumatic Diseases
University Hospitals of Cleveland

Preface

Osteoarthritis can certainly have an impact on you and your family. Make no bones about it! Upon being diagnosed, many questions may come to mind. Physicians or other professionals may be able to answer some of them. Others may not have any answers, and this can be upsetting. It can also be upsetting to realize that this is happening to *you*. Living with osteoarthritis can be very depressing, unless you learn how to think positively and make any necessary changes.

Fortunately, medical science has made a great deal of progress in treating and controlling osteoarthritis. So there is every chance that you will be able to lead a more normal and productive life. But what about the psychological effects of your condition? Will it interfere with your previous lifestyle? Will you be able to handle the pain? A major factor, then, in determining how normal and emotionally stable your life will be, is *how well you cope with osteoarthritis*.

Powerful stuff? It certainly is, but now you know why this book was written in the first place! It's filled with facts, suggestions, techniques, strategies, and other useful ideas. It was written specifically for you and for members of your family and friends.

The first part of the book presents some background information about osteoarthritis: what it is, what the symptoms are, an overview of how to treat it, and so on. The other sections deal with different aspects of living with the disease, including coping with emotions, changes in lifestyle, and living with others. These are all important aspects of coping with this or any other chronic condition. We will explore them in detail, and you'll find suggestions and strategies as well as illustrative examples for each component. In fact, a lot of the information you'll read can (and does!) apply to any chronic condition. In this book, however, the main focus is on your life with osteoarthritis.

Remember that you are a unique person. Even though a lot of similarities exist, your own life with osteoarthritis, the way it affects you, and the way you experience it will not be exactly the same as anyone else's. Therefore, it will be up to *you* to use the suggestions and strategies in this book to help you to cope as well as you possibly can. As you read about others' experiences, you'll see that you're not alone. Others feel the same way that you do, and this can be very reassuring.

Researchers are working hard, trying to find a cure for osteoarthritis. But until that time, you'll have to learn to live with it. I hope this book will be of help to you and your family. Remember: you can *always* improve the quality of your life.

Robert H. Phillips, Ph.D.
Center for Coping with Chronic Conditions
Long Island, NY

PART I.
Osteoarthritis—An Overview

1

Osteoarthritis—What Is It?

Eleanor, a 59-year-old account executive, had been feeling achy and uncomfortable for quite a while. Only recently, however, did she notice that her pain just didn't seem to be going away. In the past, she had chosen to just "live with it." But now, with the pain affecting her knees, hips, and finger joints, it hurt to even move. Finally, she took time off from work and dragged herself (painfully!) to the doctor. She received a complete physical examination, a number of blood tests, and a series of x-rays. After analyzing all the results, the doctor gently sat Eleanor down and said, "You have osteoarthritis." Marie's resigned reaction was, "Oh, no, what do I do now?"

Yes, Eleanor had osteoarthritis (OA), a chronic degenerative disease primarily affecting the joints of the body. Why is it called degenerative? Because the smooth lining that covers your bones (the cartilage) wears down (degenerates). "Osteo" means bones, so osteoarthritis literally means an inflammation of the bones in a joint. This is not totally accurate, so osteoarthritis is also called osteoarthrosis (a disease or condition affecting bones in a joint) or degenerative joint disease. We won't mention what I'm sure you'd like to call it! In order to better understand OA, let's talk a little bit about the body part most affected by this disease.

WELCOME TO THE JOINT!

"The ankle bone's connected to the shin bone; the shin bone's connected to the knee bone; the knee bone's connected to the thigh bone . . ." and so on. You may recognize these lines as the lyrics to an old ditty that you've probably sung many times. But they're not anatomically correct! The bones are not directly connected to each other. Rather, they're connected by tendons, ligaments, and muscles. The area where the bones come together forms what we know as a joint (also called an articulation), and is enclosed in a covering called the joint capsule.

What's the joint for? It permits motion. So the joint is a very important structure. Why? It's going to do a lot of hard work. Stop and think for a moment about the millions of times you move different joints in your body each day. Just today you've probably already yawned, stretched, stood up, or sat down. In addition, every time you move, it's rarely one simple joint that's moving. Usually, a number of joints are involved in any one movement. Think about how much wear and tear each of your joints will experience in your lifetime. It is remarkable to think that, for the most part, joint movement is smooth, frictionless, and painless.

Not all joints are structured the same way, nor is it necessary to go into detail concerning any of the other structures of the joint, such as the ligaments, bursa, tendons, and muscles. Rather, this discussion should serve to emphasize the structures that are important in osteoarthritis.

Cartilage

Picture the ends of the two bones that meet at a joint. They need protection so that they won't keep banging against each other, wearing each other out. So the end of each bone is covered by a smooth, white, connective tissue (up to an eighth of an inch thick) called cartilage. The cartilage creates smooth, elastic, resilient surfaces that can rub against each other with very little friction, especially when properly lubricated. What does the lubricating? No, not your local gas station mechanic. The cartilage is kept wet and moving smoothly by a substance called synovial fluid. This fluid is produced by the synovial membrane, found inside each joint capsule.

In normal cases, all parts of the joint (such as the bone, cartilage, and synovial fluid) work smoothly together. But if they don't . . . ouch!

Types of Joints

All the joints in the skeleton can be grouped into three categories, depending on the kind and degree of movement they allow. The first category is the immovable joint. The joints of the skull would be one example. The bones of the skull fit together in an interlocking pattern to protect the brain. The immovable joints are not considered to be part of the osteoarthritis discussion.

The second type of joint is the slightly movable joint. Although the joints in this category do not move very much, there is a little bit of flexibility built into the joint structure. An example of this category would be the bones of the spinal column. The bones of the spine are called vertebrae. The cartilage protecting them forms cushiony pads, called discs. Osteoarthritis can affect these joints.

The third type of joint is the movable joint. Examples include the joints of the fingers, toes, hips, ankles, and knees. These are the joints that are usually referred to when you're casually talking about your joints. They are also the ones that may be primarily involved in osteoarthritis.

WHAT CAUSES OA?

In discussing the causes of OA, it's important to mention the two main classifications of the disease: primary and secondary.

Primary osteoarthritis (also called idiopathic osteoarthritis) refers to the condition that develops for no apparent reason, other than possibly age or "wear and tear" (a description that is not totally accurate).

Secondary osteoarthritis, on the other hand, usually has more specific underlying influences. You've read, for example, about athletes who have had to retire because of the joint damage that was suffered from years of sports activities. People whose work (or even play) puts prolonged, intense pressure on the joints may develop secondary osteoarthritis. So secondary osteoarthritis might be found long after the occurrence of any number of precipitating factors, including: traumatic injury, problems with a joint (such as a fracture or infection), repeated stress to a joint (such as in athletes, ballet dancers, typists, among others), or another disease, such as rheumatoid arthritis. Being overweight could possibly cause secondary osteoarthritis! If you are overweight you'll put extra weight on your weight-bearing joints!

Although much knowledge about OA has been gained through research, the exact cause of the disease is still unknown. There are a number of factors that may play a role in the development of the disease, although that doesn't mean that any of these factors *cause* osteoarthritis. Examples? Your age, family history, medical history, and physical activities are among the factors that may be involved. One confusing issue is why some people seem to be more vulnerable to OA onset and progression than others.

WHAT EXACTLY HAPPENS IN OA?

For some reason, the cartilage protecting the bone wears away. This allows the bones to come closer together, which causes a narrowing of the joint space (as seen in x-rays). As a result, the bones in the joint rub together when you move. This can be painful. In addition, for some unknown reason, when cartilage covering bone breaks down, the end of the bone responds by getting larger! These new bone formations, also called bone spurs or osteophytes, may compound the problem and add to the pain.

HOW DOES OA OCCUR?

Unlike other chronic diseases, OA has a fairly typical pattern of symptoms. Regardless of whether you have primary or secondary osteoarthritis, or which joints are affected, the destruction of cartilage and resulting overgrowth of bone spurs usually occur in a similar manner. The one varying factor is how far these cartilage and bone changes will go.

In most cases, the onset of osteoarthritis is fairly slow. It may take months, but usually it takes years for cartilage to wear down to the point where pain occurs. But even then, there is a lot of variability in the way people experience OA. The pain can range from mild to severe. Different joints may hurt at different times. You might be in constant pain, or there may be times when you don't hurt at all. Fortunately, a majority of cases of OA are mild enough so that pain rarely exceeds a moderate level, usually occurring only after you have strenuously exerted yourself. In a smaller percentage of cases, OA can progress to the point of more intense, constant pain. Joints can sometimes be seriously affected, leading to deformity and significantly reduced mobility. Is it easy to predict how far osteoarthritis will develop in different people? Not at all!

WHAT JOINTS ARE AFFECTED?

Osteoarthritis seems to affect certain joints more than others. For example, each of your fingers has three joints: the base, the middle, and the tip. When OA spurs develop on the tip joints of your fingers, the bumps that result are called Heberden's nodes. If it affects the middle joints, the bumps are called Bouchard's nodes. Osteoarthritis is more likely to affect the tip and middle joints than the base joint, although base joints can be affected also.

Osteoarthritis usually affects weight-bearing joints. The joints most often involved are the knees and the hips. The feet and spine are affected as well. Often, joints on both sides of the body become affected, such as both hips or both knees. This is referred to as "being symmetrical." But in some cases, only a few joints may be involved in a nonsymmetrical manner.

OA can also affect the vertebrae of the spine. Damage can affect the discs, which serve as the shock absorbers, keeping the bones separated and comfortably cushioned, or bone spurs can grow on the vertebrae themselves.

Other joints that may be affected by osteoarthritis include neck, toes, and ankles (although not as often). Primary OA usually affects finger joints first, then the big toes, and then one or more of the weight-bearing joints, such as the hips and knees. Part of the spine may also be affected by primary OA. Shoulders, elbows, and wrists are less often affected by primary OA. Secondary OA rarely affects more than a few joints, and often affects only one or two joints. Most often, secondary OA affects the hip, knees, ankles, or big toe. Why? Because these are the primary weight-bearing joints of the body.

Muscles can also be affected in OA. They seem to get tired, and are unable to work as hard as they used to. This can be a problem, since strong muscles support joints and help them move. When joints are painful because of cartilage degeneration, muscles have to work harder to support joint movement. When muscles weaken, they don't help the joints as much. Also, weaker muscles lead to an unstable joint, one that wobbles. This can cause even more wear and tear, leading to more degeneration. So you can see how the joint and muscle problems of OA can cause a vicious cycle of discomfort and reduced mobility.

SYMPTOMS OF OA

Symptoms of osteoarthritis vary from person to person. What's the primary symptom of OA? Pain! It may begin as stiffness, soreness, or an aching sensation. In the early stages, pain is felt when moving or shortly afterward. Activity tends to increase the amount of pain you feel. Fortunately, rest relieves this pain! But stiffness can result from resting. (Sometimes it may seem like you just can't win!) In more advanced OA, pain may exist even if you're resting. It may become so intense that it hurts to even exercise the affected joints. Pain is an essential barometer in determining how OA is affecting you.

In addition to pain, other symptoms do occasionally occur. A noticeable sign of progressing OA is reduced mobility. You just can't move the way you used to. Why? As cartilage in certain joints break down, you'll experience more pain from joint movement. Reduced joint mobility occurs as a result of this, combined with the following: weaker, spasmodic muscles, bone spurs, or fragments in your joints.

Other signs of OA include crepitus (which is the crackling or grating noise "heard" or felt in moving joints) and joint enlargement (due to inflammation or bone changes). Heberden's nodes and Bouchard's nodes, described earlier, are also trademarks of OA.

In some cases, inflammation can occur in osteoarthritis, but it is usually mild. This may cause feelings of tenderness in the joint.

Unlike some other forms of arthritis, OA doesn't affect organs of the body, such as the heart, kidneys, or lungs. Usually, only a few joints are affected. And other common signs of illness, such as fever, changes in appetite, or feelings of malaise, are not as much a factor as they might be in inflammatory types of arthritis such as rheumatoid arthritis.

WHO GETS OA?

If you have osteoarthritis, you are certainly not alone! OA is a very common disease. It's estimated that in the United States alone, 30 to 40 million people have osteoarthritis. Although most people will have some form of OA by the time they are in their sixties or seventies, in many cases, their OA is only detected by x-ray. They may not be experiencing any symptoms, or whatever they do feel is "handleable!" But osteoarthritis is not just a "senior's" disease. Many people develop OA in their thirties and forties, some even younger, especially if there are specific secondary causes for disease onset.

Considering all ages, there seems to be a fairly equal number of men and women who develop OA. However, more men under age forty-five and more women over fifty-five develop OA. This may occur because secondary causes are more prevalent in men.

WHERE IN THE WORLD DOES OA OCCUR?

Some people feel that different types of regions may have a higher incidence of OA. In fact, some studies suggest that osteoarthritis is less prevalent in more northerly regions. But, there is no specific geographic location that is more or less prone to osteoarthritis. It seems that individuals in all parts of the world can develop OA.

Climate also seems to be of little importance. You might prefer a certain type of climate, and you may notice that you may feel more or less comfortable in different climates, but research has not yet proven that any type of climate plays a significant role in the development or progression of osteoarthritis.

2

Diagnosing Osteoarthritis

Remember Eleanor from Chapter 1? She knew she was in pain, but couldn't believe she had osteoarthritis. So she asked her doctor how the diagnosis was made.

In order for your doctor to accurately diagnose OA, any of a number of methods may be necessary, including a complete medical history, a physical examination, and x-rays. Other methods, such as blood and laboratory tests, may also be used but usually to rule out other diseases rather than to confirm a diagnosis of OA. Current symptoms and a physical examination are the most important parts of the diagnostic procedure. X-rays are usually required to confirm the physician's diagnosis and to determine how severe the OA is.

MEDICAL HISTORY

The first step in diagnosing osteoarthritis is for your doctor to get a detailed medical history from you. What are some of the more important questions? "Where are the aches and pains?" "What joints hurt?" "How long have they hurt?" "What seems to help them?" "What time of day do they bother you the most?" "Do you experience any stiffness; how long does it last?" "What injuries have you experienced to your joints?" These are among the many questions that may be asked.

PHYSICAL EXAMINATION

During the physical exam, the physician will try to determine your general state of health, as well as what specific symptoms exist. Your physician will check your joints carefully. This "investigation" will look for joints that show signs of tenderness, redness, warmth, swelling, or inflammation. Your doctor will look, touch, and listen for any kind of abnormality.

Your physician will carefully observe you as you attempt to move certain joints, focusing on any signs of crepitus (bones rubbing together within a joint). The doctor will then check your muscles for any signs of weakness or spasm. Finally, you'll be checked for other specific signs of osteoarthritis, such as Heberden's nodes or Bouchard's nodes. Often, your doctor will be able to diagnose your condition based on your family history and the findings of your physical examination.

X-RAYS

X-rays can be an important assessment tool for OA. However, they are useful only when the disease has advanced to the stage where they can actually *show* something. Earlier on, x-rays may not clearly show damage to the bones or cartilage. So why bother? Well, there's still an advantage to early x-rays. They provide a baseline against which later x-rays can be compared to see how the disease is advancing or if the illness is causing further deterioration. They can also show doctors how well treatment programs are controlling the progression of the disease. X-rays can also determine if sufficient bone damage exists to necessitate joint replacement surgery.

What do you see in x-rays? If cartilage is breaking down or has worn away in a joint, x-rays can show a narrowing within the joint space. X-rays can show the formation of new bone growths (spurs or osteophytes, which can contribute to the pain or restricted mobility of OA) and cysts. X-rays can even show bone fragments floating within the joint capsule, indicating degeneration. All of these findings, and others, can contribute to a diagnosis of OA.

ANYTHING ELSE?

There are lots of laboratory tests available, but their results are usually normal for a person with OA. If used, the purpose of the tests may be to rule out other diseases. So the primary method of diagnosing OA is the physical examination and, to a lesser degree, x-rays.

3

Treatment of Osteoarthritis

Eleanor learned a little about how OA was diagnosed from the discussion with her doctor. But even more important than this was her question, "What can you do to treat my condition?" This is the most important question for most people with OA.

Some unhappy people believe that once you have OA, you can't do much to stop it from progressing into a severely crippling, deforming, and incapacitating illness. This couldn't be further from the truth. Sure, there are a few cases where OA may continue to progress despite all therapeutic efforts. However, in most cases, a good, comprehensive treatment program can help you to live a comfortable and satisfying (if not totally pain-free) life.

How do you determine the best treatment for your OA? Unfortunately, this is usually a trial-and-error process. But you can help by understanding the disease and the way it works, and by carefully following your treatment program.

GOALS OF TREATMENT

What is the most important goal of treatment? To help you to live as normal a life as possible. How? By controlling the pain! Hopefully, treatment for OA will stabilize your condition. This is certainly a goal worth shooting for.

Why is treatment of OA so frustrating? One reason is that it has no magic cure. There's no pill that will stop the breakdown of cartilage. There's no surgical procedure that will eliminate the illness. There's no injection that will restore a joint to its original healthy condition. No treatment is 100 percent effective in controlling *all* symptoms. Since OA cannot be fully cured, it's better to consider your treatment program as more of a management program. But treatment for OA *can* be very positive and productive.

What are the general goals of treatment? There are basically four: (1) To reduce or relieve pain, (2) To preserve function, (3) To maintain or increase strength and mobility, allowing you to keep your joints functioning as smoothly and as effectively as possible, and (4) To prevent deformity. Remember: by the time you're diagnosed, your OA will have already caused damage for a long time. But your treatment program will aim to prevent further damage and to avoid deformities. Additional treatment may attempt to correct any deformities that have already occurred.

WHO PLANS YOUR TREATMENT?

Treatment programs are usually developed by a team of health care professionals, including physicians, physical therapists, occupational therapists, social workers, and rehab specialists. Initially, your physician may be the one most directly involved in planning your treatment program.

COMPONENTS OF TREATMENT PROGRAMS

Because OA can affect different people in different ways, each treatment program is individual and unique. Your own treatment program will vary, and will depend on many factors. For example, how severe is your OA? How long have you had it? Which joints are affected? Other factors such as your age, overall general health, family situation, lifestyle, and occupation will also be taken into consideration.

Most treatment programs take a sensible, conservative approach. Physicians believe that this is best for long-term progress and results. This is usually better than a very aggressive program that expects immediate spectacular results.

WHAT TREATMENT IS BEST?

Because there is no one particular treatment that is best for every person with OA, the program that you'll follow is a "package"—a combination of strategies. Your treatment program may include any or all of the following: rest, exercise, medication (to control pain and reduce inflammation), physical aids and other assistance devices, physical therapy, and other methods to control pain and improve mobility. Occasionally, surgery may be an adjunct to the treatment program. Any complete treatment program also attempts to help you deal with the emotional difficulties you may experience as a result of your OA—not just the physical difficulties.

Finally, and very importantly, treatment programs include a modified and improved long-term change in lifestyle. More detail regarding these components will be found in Part III, "Changes in General Lifestyle."

WHAT'S THE PROGNOSIS?

What is the prognosis for osteoarthritis? Doctors have a difficult time predicting how it will affect any particular individual. Fortunately, most people with osteoarthritis can be prevented from experiencing serious trouble and can continue to live satisfying, productive lives.

Is there any way of predicting whether your OA will stay the same, get better, or even get worse? Unfortunately, no. But treatment does help. The earlier you begin treatment for OA, the better the chances of helping the disease. You can help your prognosis! Make sure you seek prompt medical attention. Make sure you properly comply with your prescribed treatment!

Learn about your illness. If you learn about OA, you can fight it better. Reading books and attending courses and seminars, among other activities, will help you to gain knowledge of OA. All these activities are offered by the Arthritis Foundation. Don't be afraid to ask your doctor any questions that you have. If you are informed and educated, you'll even be able to assist your doctor in your care.

Other than your conscientious involvement, what's the most critical variable? Proper treatment! Without it, osteoarthritis can get worse. Yes, it's possible for it to progress to the point where serious deformities and disabilities occur. And, unfortunately, any bone or joint damage that occurs is irreversible. Bone damage doesn't go away. But even if your OA doesn't get worse, not following proper treatment programs can lead to your condition becoming more painful than it needs to be. So do what you can!

A FINAL NOTE

Treatment results will be slow in coming. Don't expect overnight success. However, with patience and proper adherence to a treatment program, you *can* experience improvement!

PART II.
Your Emotions

4

Coping With Your Emotions—An Introduction

How happy are you about having OA? Well, each person's emotional responses to OA are different. Even your own reactions to OA will vary from time to time. The more severe your reactions are, the more they will interfere with your ability to cope.

When first diagnosed, some people may not even react. Either it may not seem "real" to them, or it may not even bother them, because they've been living with discomfort or pain for so long. But others will go through a hard time. Emotional reactions to OA are not always rational. As a matter of fact, in many cases they may be completely irrational!

Your emotional reactions to OA may start even before treatment has begun. Usually, reactions to diagnosis of chronic diseases depend on how suddenly these conditions develop. Since OA usually develops slowly, taking months or even years, you might adjust well, since you've had plenty of time to get used to changes. On the other hand, it may be harder to adjust to secondary osteoarthritis, since it may not take as long as primary OA to develop.

FACTORS SHAPING YOUR EMOTIONAL REACTIONS

Several factors may play a role in determining how you react to OA. Keep in mind, however, that because there are so many factors, no one can predict how any person will react at any given time.

How did you generally handle problems before your osteoarthritis was diagnosed? What was your general coping style? Were you calm or nervous? Were you persistent or did you give up easily? Were you successful in coping with stress? The way you handle life's problems in general will indicate how well you will cope with OA and its treatment. How old are you? What kind of lifestyle have you enjoyed? These factors also have a bearing on how you respond emotionally. Your general physical health prior to the onset of OA also plays a role in determining your coping ability. And what about your relationships? In many cases, your emotional reactions may reflect the responses of significant people in your life. For example, if family members or friends are anxious about your medical condition, this may affect your emotional reactions.

WHICH EMOTIONAL REACTIONS?

Do you like yourself less with osteoarthritis? Has your self-image suffered? Any loss of self-esteem can have a very unpleasant effect on you. You may not feel or behave like yourself. You'll want to deal with this right away in order to return to effective, efficient functioning.

Have you felt anger because you have to go through all this? Are you angry that your joints may never be the same, and that your life may change because of this? Are you afraid of the medication you may need? Do you become depressed when you compare your present life with the way things were? Have you felt afraid of not being able to cope? Some of the most common emotional reactions in living with OA are depression, fear, guilt, and anger. Because of the importance of coping with these emotions, a separate chapter has been devoted to each of them.

MANAGING EMOTIONAL REACTIONS

Some of the ways people have learned to adjust to OA and its treatment include therapeutic intervention, support groups, and education. Because your emotions play such an important role in your life, you'll certainly want to do the best possible job controlling them. How? Let's discuss some of the most important ways.

Medical Management

Make sure you're getting the best possible medical care. If you haven't already done so, you'll want to establish a good working relationship with your physician. This involves seeing a doctor who not only has expertise in treating osteoarthritis but also is understanding and sympathetic to your emotional needs. You'll want to be sure that your physician watches your condition carefully, so that any problems that may arise can be treated promptly. Your physician must also monitor your use of medication carefully, so that it is used most effectively and any side effects are minimized.

Support Groups

Self-help or support groups can be wonderful. You'll see how others handle problems, some of which may be the same as, or at least similar to, your own. Groups provide a forum for the exchange of feelings and ideas, as well as suggestions on how to cope better. You'll see that you're not alone. This is probably the most important reason for belonging to a group. These groups are also great for your family, giving members the chance to get some support of their own. Since one of the best ways to be in control of your emotions is to have a supportive family behind you, you should encourage their participation, too.

In groups, any topics you'd like to talk about can be discussed. You may begin to share feelings more openly when you hear others talking about subjects you were previously reluctant to bring up yourself. As a result, a feeling of closeness (almost like family) develops.

By the way, there's no law that says that emotional reactions *have* to be shared with others. It's not necessary to talk them out, although this can be helpful. But these emotional reactions do need to be recognized and worked through. That's the only way to make progress.

Belonging to a national organization, such as the Arthritis Foundation, can be helpful. Such organizations bring patients and families together, and provide lots of beneficial information. They also help to expand public awareness about OA and its treatment. This will also help you with your emotions, since the more people understand what's involved with OA, the less alone and isolated you'll feel.

Medication

You'll frequently hear about medications that improve depression, anxiety, anger, and other emotional problems. Medication prescribed for these purposes is usually not addictive, so you might not be as reluctant to take it. Antianxiety medication can be helpful. So can mood elevators and antidepressants. But just remember that your doctor is the one who is in charge of medication. Don't "play with fire."

Psychological Strategies

Professional intervention may be necessary if your emotional problems are severe, or if you want to prevent them from getting worse. Having somebody to talk to can be a big help, especially with a condition like OA.

HELPING YOURSELF

Let's discuss some of the best techniques you can use to improve the way you feel.

Laugh a Little

Humor can be an amusing and effective way to deal with emotions. Whether it is hearing a joke from someone else, laughing at yourself, or creating your own jokes, humor can be a very relaxing way of dealing with a troublesome situation.

Humor works in three ways. First of all, it reduces anxiety. Laughing is a great way to release tension. Second, it can distract you from those things or feelings that are bothering you. When you're involved in something humorous, you often feel a lot better. Think back, for example, to a time when you were depressed or uncomfortable and somebody asked if you had heard a certain joke. Initially you may have been reluctant to hear it. But before long you were probably totally absorbed in the joke, wondering what the punch line would be! The fact that humor can distract you also means that it can help you to see things from a different perspective. So you may be able to look at something more objectively, which can help you to handle it more effectively.

Finally, the ability to laugh at yourself is a helpful coping strategy. It's also an important part of maturing. How well this works, however, depends on what you're going through. It's just about impossible (and probably ridiculous) to laugh at yourself while you're going through a crisis. However, as you adjust to your condition, you can better use humor as a coping strategy.

Relaxation Procedures

Relaxation is the opposite of tension. So if you learn to relax, you'll be much less tense. But relaxation procedures, by themselves, will not totally control your emotions. So why use them? Because if you're feeling more relaxed, you'll be better able to identify those problems that are affecting you, and you'll then be better able to figure out how to deal with them. Relaxation procedures, then, can be an essential first step in coping with your emotions.

How do you relax? We're talking about clinical relaxation, now—not everyday activities like reading, gardening, listening to music, or sitting in front of the television with a can of beer! There are different types of clinical relaxation procedures. For example, *progressive relaxation* is a procedure in which you learn how to relax the muscles in your body. *Hypnosis* is another relaxation procedure, as is meditation and *the relaxation response*. There's also a procedure called *imagery*, in which you picture those things in your mind that will help you to relax, thereby making it easier for you to solve problems. (More information about imagery can be found in Chapter 14, "Pain.") Books on any of these procedures are available in your local library, and can really help you to start feeling better.

Here's a quick introduction to one relaxation procedure. I call it, appropriately, the "quick release." Read the directions first and then try it. Close your eyes, take a deep breath, and hold it as you tighten every muscle in your body that you can think of—your fists, arms, legs, stomach, neck, buttocks, etc. (Obviously, don't squeeze anything that causes you pain!) Hold your breath, keeping your muscles tense, for about six seconds. Then let it out in a "whoosh," and allow the tension to drain out of your muscles. Let your body go limp. Keep your eyes closed, and breathe rhythmically and comfortably for about twenty seconds. Repeat this tension-relaxation cycle three times. By the end of the third repetition, you'll probably feel a lot more relaxed.

Pinpointing

Are you more comfortable now? Then you're ready to proceed to the next crucial step. In order to deal with anything that's upsetting you, you'll want to determine exactly what it is that's bothering you! Make a list. Then go over what you've written. In reviewing your list, you'll see that just about every item can be placed into one of two categories. The first category contains the *modifiables*, or the things (whether problems or emotions) you *can* do something about. The second category includes the *nonmodifiables*, or things you *can't* do anything about. Why separate them? Because the two categories have different implications for dealing with them.

For the first category, you'll want to figure out what strategies you can use to improve the situation. You'll plan a course of action as soon as you identify exactly what's bothering you. How about the second category? You'll still be planning strategies, but of a different kind! Where do your emotions come from? Your mind, right? Therefore, your plan for this category is to work on the way you're thinking!

What Should You Do?

How can you change the way that you think so that something will bother you less? The technique you use really depends on what emotional reaction is bothering you. For example, if you're afraid of something and you want to conquer this fear, a procedure called *systematic desensitization* may be helpful. We'll go into this later in Chapter 7 on "Fears and Anxieties."

If you're feeling guilty or angry about something, or if something is depressing you, it can be very helpful to learn how to change or "restructure" the way you're thinking. You'll learn about more techniques for that in Chapters 6, 8, and 9.

Actually, any of the procedures we've discussed can be used with just about any problem. It's just a question of deciding what's best for *you* in how to cope with your emotions.

WHAT ABOUT THE FUTURE?

Even if you do have intense emotional reactions, these will diminish, either because of the passage of time or because you're doing something to help. On the other hand, you'll experience more emotional reactions when your symptoms are more pronounced. So you'll probably experience a range of emotions from time to time. But even when these feelings do occur, you can usually point to so many positive things going on in your life—so many areas in which you can recognize progress—that it's not such a difficult thing to deal with.

Although emotions do not cause osteoarthritis, they can certainly interfere with your ability to live comfortably with the disease. So doesn't it make sense to do what you can to control your emotions?

The purpose of this section is to help you to understand the different emotions you may experience. You'll discover where they come from and, very importantly, recognize that many others have gone through exactly what you're going through. In addition, a number of strategies will be presented to help you cope with these emotions more effectively. Remember that "practice makes better." (There's no such thing as perfect!) Just reading about a method to control an emotion doesn't mean you'll experience instant success. You have to keep practicing.

In the following chapters, you'll see how these different techniques can be used. So don't be afraid, depressed, guilty, or angry! Instead, read on!

5

Coping With the Diagnosis

When you first found out you had osteoarthritis, how did you feel? How did you react when your doctor gave a name to your pain? Many people with OA, especially with primary OA, aren't terribly surprised. They may have expected that there be some medical explanation for their joints' hurting more and more. Now, at least with a name to the disease, treatment can begin in earnest (or in anyone else who has it!).

However, reactions to diagnoses of OA may not be received as well in individuals with secondary osteoarthritis, because they may not have been expecting it, and they may see it as interfering more drastically with their lifestyle. For example, athletes who develop secondary osteoarthritis may fear a premature end to their careers. Then what? Some of the more common reactions, such as anxiety, relief, and denial will be discussed in this chapter.

YOU MIGHT FEEL ANXIOUS!

What might you be thinking at the time of diagnosis? Regardless of how long your symptoms have taken to develop, you might be thinking a number of things. "I'm too young for this!" "Oh no, what's going to happen to me?" "How will the disease affect me?" "I don't want an 'old age' disease." "Will I ever be 'normal'?" "What is the treatment (and how will I handle it)?" "Am I going to be confined to a wheelchair?" "Will I ever get better?" "Who will take care of me?" "Am I going to be crippled for life?" These are all distressing questions that may pop up when you're diagnosed. Family members and loved ones may ask them as well. You may think that your life may never be the same again, for life will now include OA and its treatment.

Let's talk about this reaction. Does anyone you know like pain or physical restrictions? No way. It's normal to be afraid. You may suddenly be hit with the fact that you are mortal and vulnerable. You'll realize you may have this problem for the rest of your life. Physically, it's not uncommon to feel faint, to have a shortness of breath, or to experience other stress reactions at the time of diagnosis.

YOU MIGHT BE RELIEVED!

Does everyone feel anxious and afraid when diagnosed? Strangely, no. Some people feel relieved when diagnosed with OA! Why would you be relieved to know that you have OA? Well, perhaps you were experiencing a lot of pain and nothing seemed to help. Maybe your family and friends didn't believe you, and thought the pain was more in your head than in your joints! Maybe you thought the pain was caused by a tumor or a fatal illness (some people do actually feel this way!), and were relieved to find out that you weren't dying. Just knowing what's going on can be a relief.

There are other reasons you might be relieved after your diagnosis. First, you're probably hopeful that treatment will significantly improve the way you've been feeling (and it's good to finally know *why* you're feeling that way). Second, family members and friends who may not have believed that you were really in pain will now discover the truth. Unfortunately, some people close to you may still not believe that the problem is physical. They may continue to believe that the problem is either emotional or stress-related. You can't force everyone to believe a medical diagnosis! However, most doubts will probably disappear, and strained relationships may improve. Family members may sometimes feel guilty as they realize that they have been skeptical about your condition. They may have criticized your inability to fulfill responsibilities and your decreased ability to do things. They did this because they thought a real illness did not exist. Now they will know the truth! Third, and most important, you'll be relieved that *it wasn't all in your head*. After a long period of time, even the most confident person can begin to wonder if there is really something wrong or if the problem is purely emotional.

HOW ABOUT DENIAL?

Denying that a problem exists is not unusual. Regardless of what symptoms you've been experiencing, hearing that you have OA may provoke denial. You might be willing to deal with the symptoms, but not with having a permanent label attached to them. So you may protest, "Oh, you're just making that up," "I don't have this problem the way you think I do," "Why don't you give it a little more time; I'm sure the problem will go away by itself," or even "#!(*)x#—leave me alone!"

If you're reading this book, then chances are you're probably not denying your condition. But if you *are* denying it, the best way to start coping with your situation is to face reality. Speak to those professionals who know about your condition, and have them explain it in further detail. Let them explain why treatment is necessary. Look at any x-rays that have been taken. Talk to other people with OA, and listen to what they experienced in the earlier stages of their disease. You will find that many of their stories are similar to your own. You may also discover self-help groups that can add to your knowledge of OA, as well as your coping ability.

Did you ever ask yourself, "Why can't things go back to the way they used to be?" Have you ever wished you could wake up one morning and find out that this was all a bad dream? The more you keep hoping that it will go away, the more you are slowing down your adjustment. Why is this so? Because you're not really admitting to yourself that you have changed—perhaps permanently. Rather, you're trying to push it out of your mind, hoping that things will return to the way they were. Such denial can obviously make it hard to cope with having OA, since the problem is not being faced realistically. Try to recognize that your condition does exist now, that it affects you, and that it will remain with you. Try to plan all your activities and aim all your thinking toward the notion that you are going to do what you can to handle it effectively.

DEATH WISH

Have you ever wished you could die since being told you have OA? Some people do. Emotionally, they exclaim that they'd rather die than have to go through this. They feel their joints are only going to deteriorate more, the pain is only going to get worse, and there will be more and more things they can't do, so why bother living? If you've ever felt this way, don't feel guilty about such thoughts. You're not alone. Although you may feel like giving up from time to time, these feelings can and will go away if you work hard enough on them. And think of all the positive things you *still* can enjoy in your life!

HOW DO YOU START TO ADJUST?

You must help yourself. Sure, you can receive love and support from your family and friends, and you can get expertise and support from professionals. But that's never enough. *You* are the one who is going to have to come to grips with your condition. This is something you have to do yourself, regardless of what anyone else says or does. At first, adjusting may be a very difficult and ongoing struggle. It may require a lot of effort and understanding. You may go through a lot of emotional turmoil, but there is no other way. You must face it.

Information, please! Get as much of it as you can. If you had trouble accepting your diagnosis, it was probably because you didn't know enough about OA. So you'll want to learn as much as possible. Your physician will be helpful in providing information, or will at least suggest ways of getting it. Read a lot, but make sure that your reading material is current.

After reading general, consumer-oriented information, you might want to move on to more technical material. Ask questions about anything you don't understand. It probably wasn't a lifelong goal of yours to become an expert on OA, but think about how much this can help you. Doctors will respect your questions more. And you'll understand exactly what's going on in your joints. These are just two of the many advantages that can come from reading about your condition.

Organizations such as the Arthritis Foundation have the specific purpose of providing you with current information on OA. Not only does the Arthritis Foundation have reading material, but it sponsors forums, symposia, speakers, arthritis clubs, and arthritis self-help classes all designed to help you.

Beware of Less Reputable Sources

Should you believe everything you read? Of course not. You may come across "cures" in weekly newspapers or magazines that sound incredible—alternatives for proper treatment that make you regret having started them in the first place. Or you may read in a glossy, weekly magazine that wearing a chestnut on your body is successful in stopping the pain of OA! (*Nuts* to that idea!) Make sure that whatever you read is reputable, and remember that it takes rigorous scientific study before one can prove that a new procedure or treatment is actually effective. And be sensible. If some exciting new treatment or medication were discovered, wouldn't you expect to learn about it in your daily newspaper or on a national news program? More about this later in Chapter 22, "Quackery."

Dealing With Your Emotional Reactions

Begin working consciously to control any anxiety or stress that's making you feel less than comfortable. Once you have accepted the fact that you have a chronic medical condition and will have to alter your lifestyle, you'll want to try to control as many harmful emotions as you can.

It's very easy for your imagination to run wild. You'll probably keep thinking about all the things that can possibly go wrong. You'll worry about every joint. So learn the facts about your condition. This is a great way to alleviate some of the anxiety caused by the diagnosis.

The emotions stemming from any chronic condition can be unpleasant. You may engage in prolonged periods of regret, sorrow, and nostalgia, remembering the way it used to be. Many fears will come to mind, some of which can be overwhelming. Fear of incapacitation, of being handicapped, of losing out on life—all are very understandable fears. Begin facing them. They can and must be faced in order to move your adjustment along more smoothly. Speak to other people who have OA. Learn how they've adjusted. This can be very helpful.

WHAT'S NEXT?

Once you've become more familiar with your condition, and understand how it affects you, what can you do to deal with it? For one thing, learn what specific changes may have to be made in your lifestyle. There is no way of knowing how many changes you'll have to make, but you do want to create the best possible life for yourself.

Obviously, work with a physician you can trust, one who has had previous experience working with people with OA. You want to find a physician you feel comfortable with. Remember that the patient-physician relationship you develop now will be helpful throughout your life with OA.

How About the Family?

If your family can learn how to cope with your diagnosis, you will adjust much more easily. It's hard for everyone if those around you have difficulty accepting your condition. But dealing with the diagnosis can be hard for family members. They, too, will go through periods of denial when they will say, "No, everything will be fine," or "I'm sure the problem will clear up by itself."

Loretta, a 56-year-old receptionist, had only recently been diagnosed as having OA. After a few depressing weeks, however, she began to learn how to cope. She was finally able to handle thoughts of lifestyle changes, concerns about reduced mobility, and some of the other unpleasant thoughts associated with OA. Sound great? Not really. You see, her husband of thirty-seven years couldn't face having a wife who couldn't do what she used to do, her children were afraid she was going to become more dependent on them, and her 82-year-old mother was having a hard time dealing with the guilt. Although Loretta was learning how to cope with OA, she could not cope with her family. They couldn't handle it, and were making things very difficult for her.

It's a great idea for family members to seek out people to speak to. They, too, can find out more about OA and about how others cope with treatment. Family members can follow the same suggestions given before: seeking self-help groups, speaking to physicians, and reading. So encourage family members and any willing friends to learn as much as they can. This will help your adjustment.

IN A NUTSHELL

Start thinking positively about your life with OA. Learn as much as you can about your condition. Use whatever support systems are necessary to help you. Use all the stress management and emotional control procedures available. Start saying to yourself, "OA may be affecting me, but I'm still alive and I'm going to do whatever I can to help myself adjust to this." If it's necessary for you to make changes in your lifestyle, even major ones, tell yourself that you will make them, and that you will make them willingly! You are going to lead as complete a life as you can. The more quickly you can adapt your lifestyle to fit your needs, the more rapidly you will be able to enjoy your life. This may be hard at first and will take time. But at least be grateful that you're not helpless and can take steps to make the most of your life with OA!

6

Depression

Sam was depressed. He was a 64-year-old man who had successfully raised three children, been married for forty-four years, and lived in a beautiful home in a well-to-do neighborhood. It looked as though he had everything he could ever ask for—except a life without OA! And oh, what an effect this had on him! In the past, Sam had always been enthusiastic about life. But he now became extremely unhappy whenever he thought about the future. He felt that he couldn't get around the way he used to, and was afraid he would end up confined to a wheelchair. He didn't even want to spend time with his children or grandchildren. Yes, Sam was suffering from depression.

Depression is a serious problem. The very mention of the word can sometimes knock the smile right off your face. Actual numbers vary, but it is estimated that more than two million Americans need professional care for depression. Because it is so widespread, depression has been nicknamed the "common cold" of emotional problems.

Just what is depression? Depression is an extremely unpleasant feeling of unhappiness and despair. It can range from mild (where you may feel discouraged and downhearted) to severe (where you can feel utterly hopeless, worthless, and unwilling to go on living). You may feel that there is no reason to remain a part of the world.

Depression can be painful. Imagine how it must hurt to feel (or say), "I wish I were never born. What good am I? I'm not helping anybody around me and I'm not helping myself." It may seem like life and the world are against you. Life may seem unfair—a constant struggle in which you never win. That hurts.

DEPRESSION AFFECTS YOUR BODY

The more noticeable symptoms of depression may be physical. Nervous activity or agitation, such as wringing of the hands, may occur. You may be restless, or have difficulty remaining in one place. On the other hand, you may become much less active, and remain motionless for abnormally long periods of time (appearing as if you are almost in a trance, with no apparent desire to do anything). Sam's wife, Helen, became very concerned when her husband remained seated in a chair in the living room for hours at a time. When she asked him a question, he would respond in monosyllables. When friends called on the phone, he never wanted to talk to them. Sam's depression was causing him to lose interest in just about everything.

Other physical changes that can occur are a reduction or increase in appetite, a decreased interest in sex, and, for some women, cessation of menstruation. If you're mildly depressed, you may have difficulty concentrating, and you attention span may be much shorter. Guys may remain unshaven simply because they don't feel like shaving. When you speak (and you'll probably do less of that, too), your conversation will usually be shallow, emphasizing feelings of worthlessness and despair. Most of your physical activities will also slow down (and not just because of OA restrictions).

You'll probably feel exhausted. This may seem surprising, since you're not doing much of anything anyway. But constantly telling yourself that you're no good can be very tiring! You really don't want to believe this, but you feel like you have no choice. In attempting to escape these feelings, you may become even more depressed, as well as more physically drained and exhausted.

There are many ways that your body may react when you're depressed. Depression may cause you to feel physically sick. Any of the symptoms we've talked about thus far might be related to a physical disorder. But if the symptoms go away when your depression improves, don't just assume that they're related to the depression. A medical examination may still be a good idea. This way, you'll be sure that there is no organic disease causing your depression.

DEPRESSION AFFECTS YOUR MOOD

You may experience frequent mood swings. For example, you might feel worse in the morning and better in the evening. This may be because of joint stiffness and pain, as well as depression. Another reason why you may feel better in the evening is that you realize it's almost time to go to sleep—a means of escape. But depression may also cause difficulty sleeping, even if you weren't doing much of anything during the day.

When you're depressed, you may feel like your mood keeps getting "lower." You may like yourself very little, if at all. Your thinking may be very negative—very different from the way it is when you're feeling good.

It is your negative thinking (not just a particular triggering event) that leads to your depression. This negative thinking tends to be the most frequently overlooked and misunderstood part of depression. Recognizing this is an important first step in learning to cope with depression.

DEPRESSION AFFECTS RELATIONSHIPS WITH OTHERS

If you're depressed, you may feel that people around you have no need for you. As Sam used to complain, "Why should my friends want to see me or make plans with me? I can't do anything!"

Do you feel less at ease talking to others? Does it seem as if others are having a hard time talking to you, even if they have been close to you for a long time? Because of your depression, you may be less interested in conversation and less confident. You may project *your* feelings of self-worthlessness onto others, believing that they really don't want to talk to you. The more depressed you are, the more persuasive you may be in convincing other people around you that you are no good.

Ann received a telephone call from her friend Regina. Regina wanted to know how Ann had been feeling, since the last time they had gotten together Ann had seemed to be in a great deal of pain. Ann responded halfheartedly, sensing that Regina was only calling out of obligation. She then explained that she would understand if Regina did not want to call again, since she never seemed to have any good news to tell her. How do you think Regina felt? Imagine hearing this repeatedly, despite having reassured Ann that her concern was sincere. Would you be surprised if, eventually, Regina got tired of even trying, and stopped calling? But in Ann's mind, this would only reinforce the fact that she really was no good, and that she was not worthy of having any friends after all!

DEPRESSION AFFECTS PHYSICAL ACTIVITIES

Do you find that you are getting less satisfaction from your normal activities? Are you functioning like a robot? Does it seem as if something is missing? It can be depressing to realize that something you used to enjoy no longer gives you the same pleasure, especially if you don't know why. It almost seems as if there is a force propelling you to "go through the motions," while your heart just isn't in it. It is understandable, therefore, that if you are depressed, you might prefer to withdraw from such activities. What happens after that first depressing event occurs? A kind of chain reaction follows. This one occurrence creates a feeling that spreads like wildfire. It's almost as if the bottom has dropped out of your world. You may feel less able to control your thinking (although this is not true, as we will see later). But keep in mind that the deeper you go into depression, the harder it is to climb back out again. Therefore, you certainly want to catch these feelings of depression as early as possible, to try to keep yourself from spiraling further downward.

WHAT CAUSES DEPRESSION?

Why do we experience depression? Sometimes we can figure this out, and sometimes we can't. But before we give up, let's discuss some of the possible causes.

How About the Normal "Downs"?

A certain amount of depression is normal in anyone's life. Nobody's life is a constant "upper." We all experience normal cycles of ups and downs. If we never experienced some of the downs, how could we ever fully appreciate the ups?! However, when depression becomes more than just the "normal downs," then it must be attended to. Nipping it quickly in the bud can keep it from becoming much worse.

There are certain things in anyone's life that can understandably lead to depression. Certain traumatic experiences such as losing a loved one, being diagnosed with a chronic illness, requiring major surgery, or being fired from a job—all may certainly lead to depression. That would be understandable. However, this *doesn't* mean you should ignore the problem or wait until it goes away. It's essential to learn how to deal with depression, since this is so important in learning how to cope with OA.

How About Anger You Can't Express?

What if you get so angry that you feel as if you're going to burst? But you don't (or can't) do anything about it, so you decide to "swallow" it. It seems strange that a powerful feeling like anger can turn into a withdrawn, helpless feeling like depression. But it's true. If you become increasingly angry about something and feel unable to do anything about it, you may turn the anger inward. You may feel so much frustration or hopelessness that you "shut down" in an attempt to keep yourself from these terrible feelings. This leads to withdrawal, which is a symptom of depression.

Is It All in Our Minds?

A small percentage of depression cases may be caused by biochemical deficiencies—some chemical imbalance in our bodies. This does not occur very often, however. Treatment for biochemical deficiencies may involve the administration of drugs in an effort to balance the chemicals in our bodies. This usually isn't the whole answer. But regardless of whether your depression is caused by this or, more typically, by your reactions to things, people, and events around you, you should still try to modify your behavior and improve your thinking. Many experts believe that even if the cause of depression *is* biochemical, you *can* have a positive effect on your depression by working on improving your thoughts and behavior.

How About Osteoarthritis?

Can OA cause depression? Are you kidding?! Living with OA can certainly create depression or magnify already existing depression.

You may be saying to yourself, "If I'm depressed over my OA, how can I expect to get over my depression unless I can get rid of this disease?" That kind of thinking will get you nowhere. Even if your pain does totally go away, you still can't ignore the fact that your OA is a chronic condition. So if your depression lingers, don't wait. Work on it. Learn how to cope with it. We'll talk more later about how you can improve your thinking.

What else about OA might depress you? You might become depressed thinking about the future, not knowing what your prognosis is or how it will affect your life. Knowing that you need (or may need) supportive devices can be depressing, as well as the fact that you'll probably need medication to deal with the pain. Changes in habits necessitated by your condition and its treatment may also be depressing.

Problems involving other people may depress you. You may feel helpless because you are unable to share what you're experiencing or the way you feel. You may get depressed if others don't understand what you're going through. You may be depressed about the possibility of damaged relationships, lost friendships, or family friction.

WHAT MAINTAINS DEPRESSION?

You may be blaming yourself (or your OA) for everything that is wrong. You may tend to become more and more withdrawn, and pull away from the world around you. Why? Well, if you believe that your condition is causing all these horrible things, isn't it better to "escape" and not think about it? Realistically, escaping doesn't solve anything. But if you're depressed, you may feel that withdrawal is the only way to solve this dilemma. Actually, it's not the answer and may make you even more depressed.

Although you may seem sullen and withdrawn to others, you're probably in deep emotional pain. Part of what makes you, and keeps you, depressed is your failure to protect yourself from this emotional pain. When your mind does allow any thoughts to enter, you tend to feel overwhelmed by feelings of doom and destruction. You feel that nothing good can possibly happen—that only bad things can happen. So what do you do? You try to block everything out of your mind!

So why do you stay depressed? Why doesn't it just go away? It may be that you don't want to talk to anybody or even consider therapy. Therefore, the thoughts and feelings leading to your depression tend to be kept hidden. You may ask, "Is my unwillingness to talk the only reason why I'm still depressed? If I start talking more, will that get me out of my depression?" Not necessarily. But it can be helpful to talk out your feelings. It would probably be helpful (even though you wouldn't be too thrilled) if a close friend or family member took the initiative and engaged you in some kind of conversation (therapeutic or otherwise) or, at least, into doing something physical.

HOW DO WE DEAL WITH DEPRESSION?

Can anything be done? Of course! Would I abandon you without any suggestions? First, tell yourself that the *main* reason you're still depressed is that you have not yet taken the proper steps toward feeling better! These steps can "bring you out of the rut" and reacquaint you with the more positive, pleasant aspects of living that you'd like to experience. Don't think it's easy, though. Unfortunately, once you've fallen into depression, it takes effort, hard work, and a certain amount of persistence to pull yourself back up. The fight, however, is surely worth it. Of course, the fight can be made easier if you know of specific techniques and activities that will help.

Once you feel better, you're not going to ever want to feel that depressed again, right? Well, the strategies and techniques that are most effective in dealing with depression can also be effective in preventing you from becoming depressed again! This doesn't mean that you'll *never* feel depressed again. It may happen. Anticipate it, so that if it does recur, you won't completely fall apart. And if it does happen, won't it be good to know that you can fight it? You *can* do something to help yourself!

Depression Treatment

Now that you're ready to fight your depression, consider two major ways of dealing with it: being more active (in other words, *doing* something) and working on your thinking.

It can be very helpful to make a list of all the things that are depressing you. You may feel there'll be at least fifty items! But, in actuality, you'll probably start running dry after six or seven. Then divide this list into two more lists: first, things that you *can* do something about, and second, things you *can't* do anything about. (Sound familiar? You read about this earlier in the section. But it really works for a number of different problems.) Get physical (do something) about those items in the first list, and get thoughtful (work on your thinking) regarding those items in the second list.

Let's Get Physical

Unknowingly, you may be using a lot of energy to keep yourself depressed. You may be working hard to keep that anger inside, even if it appears to others that you are withdrawing. If your depression is anger turned inward, then we can logically assume that by releasing it, feelings of depression can be eliminated. But what do you do with those feelings? You must find an object toward which your anger can be expressed. This may be difficult. However, it's important to release the trapped anger so that it doesn't build up further and deepen the depression.

Have you ever been in this situation? You're sitting somewhere, depressed and withdrawn. Somebody makes an innocent remark, and you practically snap the person's head off! What's happening? Whatever was said triggered the release of the internalized anger that was making you depressed. Look out, world!

Consider for a moment all the energy that is keeping you depressed. You've read about why it is important to release this energy. What kinds of activities can be helpful for this? Many types of intense physical activity can release this energy. But although being active can make you feel better, it's your thoughts that can make you depressed. Physical activity can provide a great distraction, which can help you to look more objectively at what's going on. That will help. But it may not teach you what you need the most: ways of fighting inappropriate thinking. Besides, OA may not even allow you to participate in intense physical activity! Fortunately, this isn't the only way to lift depression.

Let's Get Thoughtful

So if you can "think" yourself into depression, you can obviously "think" yourself out of it. How? Your thoughts show how you "talk to yourself." In fact, when it comes to talking to yourself, you're probably the biggest chatterbox you know! But if you're depressed, you're just talking yourself down. All your comments (or at least most of them) are probably put-downs—harsh statements offering little to be happy about. These can make you feel even worse. You want your inner voice to help you, not hurt you. Let's see how you can do that.

Distinguishing Fact From Fiction

Don't get defensive when I tell you that when you're depressed, you tend to distort reality. Clinical research with depressed patients has proven this. Recognize, therefore, that your thoughts are not necessarily based on what is really going on, but on your own distorted views. This is called *cognitive distortion*.

Is that bad? You bet your happiness it is. "Cognitive" refers to your thinking. "Distortion" means you're twisting things around and, in general, losing sight of what's real. We all tend to do this from time to time. But when you're depressed, you do it a lot, if not all the time, and it *keeps* you depressed. So how do you stop? First, you must become reacquainted with what is really happening, and with the facts. But how can you do that if you keep distorting reality. Right now, you're better off accepting somebody *else's* perceptions of the situation, because that person is probably a lot more objective and accurate. Since so many feelings of worthlessness are based on distorted facts, depression can be reduced, if not eliminated, once these facts are straightened out.

Ella kept moaning because none of her friends were calling her. "They don't call as much as they used to. I guess they just don't care." Her daughter, Arlene, asked her to estimate how often her friends used to call. When Ella compared this number to the current number of calls she was receiving, she realized that the numbers were almost the same. She then realized that she was probably just more sensitive because of all the changes going on in her life! Although she did not feel 100 percent better, it was good to know that she wasn't being abandoned.

Making Molehills out of Mountains

Does this imply that if you're depressed you have no real problems? Is it "all in your head"? No. Everyone has problems. If you feel good, you can handle them, but if you're depressed, you may feel overwhelmed. Each and every part of your life, regardless of how trivial or slight it may be, tends to depress you. As the depression lifts, you will again be able to deal with all of life's problems—big and small.

Self-Fulfilling Prophecy

We've discussed several different ways that you may feel if you're depressed. Are all of these feelings irrational and untrue? No. Ironically, although some of them may start off being far from the truth, the longer you feel that way the more chance there will be for them to become "self-fulfilling prophecies." In other words, you'll begin convincing yourself that nonsense makes sense. For example, if you begin telling yourself that friends and relatives don't care, this may become a reality because your negative attitudes may alienate the people close to you. They may decide it's not worth the bother. As far as your activities go, you are less likely to do anything when you're depressed. You'll probably be less likely to even attempt doing things that you used to enjoy. As a result, you'll feel less competent and will not accomplish anything. This may just magnify and confirm your feelings of worthlessness, leading to even greater depression. Not a pretty picture.

Once you begin feeling depressed, your negative thoughts will soon lead to negative actions. These negative actions will lead to more negative thoughts, which will in turn lead to more negative actions, and so on. It is an ongoing, vicious circle that will spiral you further downward into deeper depression. Eventually you'll feel trapped in this vicious circle, with no way to escape from the "dumps."

Are you getting depressed just reading this? In all probability, if you've ever been depressed, you've said to yourself at least once already, "Wow, that sounds just like me!" So you see, your negative thoughts become self-fulfilling prophecies. If you find that you are starting to believe in your negative thoughts, stop yourself. Try to think positive thoughts, so that if your thought *does* turn out to be real, it will at least be a positive one.

Positive Is the Opposite of Negative

As we've said before, depression results from—and causes—a lot of negative thinking. Negative thoughts automatically pop into your mind and you cannot stop them. It's like trying to keep your eyes open when you sneeze! You just can't do it. But once you become aware of these thoughts, then you *can* do something. People who remain depressed feel incapable of doing anything about their negative thinking and allow these thoughts to continue. They simply continue in that vicious, downward circle that was mentioned earlier.

Anna was resting when the telephone rang. "I'm sure that's Kate, calling to cancel our lunch plans," she thought to herself. Within the thirty seconds it took her to get to the phone, she had become so depressed that she considered not even answering the call! Imagine how she felt when she reluctantly answered the phone and discovered that it was a wrong number! Anna had allowed her negative thoughts to run wild—she became more and more negative until she was about ready to give up. And for what? There was no clear-cut reason for thinking the way she did.

Once she realized that she was thinking this way, what should she have done? She should have *countered* her thoughts. She should have told herself, "It may not even be Kate on the phone. Or if it is, maybe she's just calling to confirm. I won't let it bother me now. After all, I don't even know who it is!" This is the beginning of positive thinking.

Dwell on the Brighter Tomorrows

If you find yourself unhappily comparing your present life to life before OA, try to modify your thinking. Start planning fun things for the present and future. You can come up with some enjoyable things to do, regardless of how restricted you may be. But it takes effort. Don't wallow in self-pity, because that will allow your depression to strangle you. Work on your thinking, develop some positive plans, and translate them into pleasure. Then wave good-bye to your depression!

When you recall the past, you may not even think it was that much better. You may have had other physical problems. You may have made some mistakes in your life. Your past may make you even more depressed about the future. However, you can't change the past. What's done is done. Keep telling yourself that. Tell yourself that you're going to work on making the future better. Set up some specific goals, starting with the easy-to-reach ones. You'll be helping yourself just by thinking about what you can do that's more positive. Don't punish yourself for the past.

What's Missing From Your Life?

You may have laughed when you read the title of this section. "Good joints," you might respond. "Mobility without pain!" Sure. But why discuss this? Because depressed people frequently lament the fact that something is missing from their lives. What is usually missing is a feeling of satisfaction, accomplishment, and pride that normally comes from others' praise. You may just miss the attention and interest of other people. This may cause you to feel worthless. How do you counteract this? Think about your positive qualities (yes, you do have some!). Think about how you can interact more with people, spark their interest, and obtain more of the satisfaction that makes you feel worthwhile.

Shoot for the Earth, Not the Moon

We all have goals for ourselves. It's normal to become depressed when we don't reach a particular goal, especially if we've tried very hard to get there. But maybe it's not a realistic goal. Maybe you're trying to do something you can't, and you're getting depressed instead of realistically resetting your goal.

Bill had not returned to work since his hip replacement surgery. Finally, after a long period of rest and rehabilitation, he was feeling better. His OA was stable, and he was looking forward to getting back to work so that he could catch up on everything. When his doctor finally gave him the "go ahead," he practically flew to his office.

After two hours of phone calls, consultations, dictation, and meetings, he was exhausted. His spirits plummeted. He became worried that he'd never again be able to handle all the pressure, and that he was in danger of losing his job. Wrong! Bill had simply set his sights too high. Expecting to return to his old schedule as if he didn't have OA was just not realistic. Try to return to your old activities slowly. Build up your stamina. Isn't the result more important? And if your goals are more realistically set, you'll have a much better chance of achieving them, and less of a chance of falling short.

AN ANTIDEPRESSING SUMMARY

The best way to work on negative thoughts is to prevent them from continuing. Try to be more positive. Deal with reality the way it actually exists. Deal with thoughts from a more factual point of view. Deal with them the way somebody else might—somebody who is not depressed and who can be more objective. Try to make your perceptions more accurate, your awareness more realistic, and your thoughts more positive and constructive. Remember: Your thoughts lead to your emotions. If your thoughts are negative and critical, then your emotions will also be in bad shape. If you can turn your thoughts around to a more positive, constructive point of view, you'll see that your emotional reactions will improve as well.

7

Fears and Anxieties

Don't be "afraid" to read this chapter! It may help you discover what you're "anxious" about!

The two sentences above may help you to distinguish between fear and anxiety. What's the difference? *Anxiety* is a general sense of uneasiness—a vague feeling of discomfort. It is an agitated, uncertain state in which you just don't feel at peace or in control. There is a premonition that something bad may happen that you have to protect yourself against. You feel very vulnerable. However, you're not exactly sure what the source of your anxiety is.

Fear, on the other hand, is usually more specific. It's often directed toward something that can be recognized, whether it's a person, object, situation, or event. We may be fearful when we become aware of something dangerous, or when we feel threatened. When we are afraid (as with feeling anxious), we also feel out of control and less confident. So the feelings of fear and anxiety are basically the same. The main difference is whether you can identify the source of the feeling. From this point on, however, I'll be using the two terms interchangeably so that there is less confusion.

Fear is so prevalent that many words are used to describe it: scared, concerned, alarmed, worried, uptight, nervous, edgy, shaky. Then there's perplexed, wary, frightened, helpless, frustrated. Is that it? Nope! How about suspicious, keyed-up, impatient, giddy, hesitant, apprehensive, tense, panicky, disturbed, agitated? Of course, there are more, but if I went on this book would have to be renamed "The Fear Synonym Book." All these words mean the same thing: "I'm afraid." The source of this fear may be real or imaginary.

IS FEAR GOOD OR BAD?

Believe it or not, fear is usually good! Now you're probably saying, "If I'm shaking with fear, how can it be good?" Fear mobilizes you. It "tells" you to prepare to attack the source of your fear. You react in a way that leads to action. In this regard, fear is similar to stress. It serves a necessary and critical purpose. In a way, it "protects" you.

Fear is bad only if it is denied, or if it is so excessive that you can't do anything about it. If you face it, push past it, and try to resolve it, then fear is a positive emotion. It is only when the source of fear becomes overlooked, ignored, or denied that the consequences may be a problem. This is because the threat or danger is allowed to continue, and nothing (or not enough) is being done to control it.

HOW INTENSE ARE OUR REACTIONS?

Fear ranges in intensity from mild to severe. It is impossible to measure how much fear there is in anyone's life. It is unique and varies from person to person.

What determines how fearful you get? Usually the strength of the feared object, person, or event is important. Also important is how close it is (wouldn't you be more afraid of getting an injection within the next thirty seconds than getting it in thirty days?); how vulnerable you are (do you *hate* injections, or are you just tired of feeling like a pincushion?); and how successful you are in conducting yourself (can you calmly accept the needle, or do you scream a lot?). These are some of the factors determining how you handle fear. Your own strength and the success of your defense mechanisms also play a role.

People with osteoarthritis can be afraid of many things. Obviously, the more fears you have, the more these can interfere with your adjustment. Recognizing your fears and learning how to deal with them will help you live more happily and more comfortably. How? I was afraid you'd never ask!

HOW TO COPE WITH FEARS AND ANXIETIES

The first step in coping with your fears is to use the "pinpointing" technique discussed in Chapter 4. List all the things you're afraid of. Identify exactly what you are afraid of and exactly why you are afraid. Then think about what you can do to alleviate your fears.

For Ruth, this was not hard. She knew she was afraid of how people would react when they saw her hands. She quickly realized that what she feared was rejection. She was concerned that they wouldn't want to be with her because of their own fears ("Could this happen to me?"). She planned a course of action (no, not a one-way ticket to Brazil!). She decided she'd simply do the best she could, expecting her friends to accept her the way she was. If they didn't, that was *their* loss. She was less afraid almost instantly. As you begin planning your strategies, and gradually put your plan into operation, you'll continue to feel better and better.

Desensitize Yourself

A great technique used to conquer fear is called *systematic desensitization*. You learn to desensitize yourself, to make yourself less vulnerable to the source of your fear.

Here's how to try it. Sit in a comfortable chair and relax. Then create a movie in your mind. Imagine what it is that makes you afraid. If you get tense, stop imagining it and relax. When you've calmed down, try imagining it again. The more you try to imagine your fear, the less it will bother you. Try it! It will give you a great feeling of relaxation and control. There are several library books that provide more information on systematic desensitization. Check them out.

It was stated earlier that anxiety is a vague, uneasy feeling with an unknown source. So how can you cope with it by following the steps listed above? Well, if you try to pinpoint the source and are unable to, then you probably can't follow the steps. So what do you do? Use relaxation procedures. Work on changing your thinking. Even if you can't pinpoint a specific fear, these techniques will greatly help you to cope with general anxiety.

LET'S TALK ABOUT SPECIFICS

Remember, it is understandable for you to have many fears related to your condition. A problem arises, however, when you don't admit these fears. As a result, you can't do anything about resolving them. They *can* be resolved. And you can work on changing your thinking.

Initial Fears

When you were first diagnosed, many fearful questions probably came to mind. "What will the future be like? What will become of me? Will I need a wheelchair? Will I be crippled?" These are all understandable questions and justifiable fears. But time goes on.

Some of these questions have been answered, and some of your initial qualms have not materialized. But you're probably still afraid of some things. Let's discuss some of them.

Fear of Pain

Nobody likes pain. Pain is probably the most unpleasant problem associated with OA. You may be afraid of pain. This fear may be just as strong when you don't have pain, since you're afraid of it happening! If you do feel pain, you'll wonder when you're going to feel some relief. You may fear each little twinge of pain, interpreted as a sign that your condition is deteriorating or that additional problems exist or may develop. What can you do about this fear? Try to accept the fact that you may always have pain, but medication can reduce its intensity. Recognize that you can do much of what you like to do, even if you're a little less comfortable. Further suggestions will be offered in Chapter 14, "Pain."

Fear of Medication and Possible Side Effects

You may be nervous about the different medications that you have to take, even though you need them. You may be afraid of what they're doing to your body. Just keep reminding yourself what your OA would be like without medication! Your physician is aware of the possible side effects, but will still prescribe medication as long as the advantages of the medication outweigh the side effects.

Fear of "What Next?"

What will happen next? You can't be sure. Will there be an increase in the amount of pain? Will new joints be affected? Will you develop new side effects from your medication? Will you need joint replacement surgery? Fear of "what next?" includes being afraid of new problems, or the return of old ones.

Everyone *wonders* what's in store for the future. But because of the OA, you may be *afraid* of the future, rather than merely curious. What can you do? Unless you own a crystal ball, you can't foresee what will happen in the future. So take life one day at a time. What will be, will be. (What a great idea for a song!) Just tell yourself that you'll handle any problems as they occur.

Fear of Disability

The thought of being disabled may be horrible. Because OA can be physically restricting, you may share this fear. But "disabled" is a bad term, since it suggests that you can't do anything. If you look around you and think more objectively, you'll realize that having a physical disability won't make you any less of a human being. You will still have many, many capabilities. Numerous Olympic champions began their athletic careers to overcome physical disabilities. Beethoven wrote some of his greatest music after becoming totally deaf. Mickey Mantle played some of his best baseball despite arthritis-related pain. And "Broadway" Joe Namath had such problems with his knees that his football career was agonizing, although highly successful! So regardless of any restrictions from OA, be assured that you can overcome or at least compensate for a limitation in one area by developing or enjoying abilities in another.

How might a disability affect you? Maybe you'll be afraid of becoming increasingly dependent on others, since you can't do as much for yourself. But it's your *thinking* that's making you afraid. Other than trying to take good care of yourself, what else can you really do? Take things as they come, but think more positively. Remember: You still have lots of room for self-fulfillment.

If you are already physically restricted, this can certainly be frightening, especially if you enjoy independence. You don't want to be a burden to those important people in your life. Can you do anything to prevent this? That depends on the nature of your restriction. Find out everything you can about the possibility of rehabilitation. If there's any chance, take advantage of it. Even if there's no possibility of total rehabilitation, every little bit helps. Regardless, remember that you'd help someone you love if it were necessary. And the important people in your life care about you, don't they? So don't let yourself give up or you'll be doing yourself an enormous disservice.

Fear of Being Crippled or in a Wheelchair

Fear of being crippled crosses the minds of most people with OA at one time or another. But be assured that a great majority of the people with OA will *not* become crippled, even if they are not able to do as much as they used to do.

Just as unlikely are your chances of ending up in a wheelchair. This would happen only if your joints were very severely damaged (and this probably is because you were neglecting your self-care). Advances in modern medicine continue to decrease the chances of being crippled or ending up in a wheelchair. (This doesn't mean that on a trip to a place like Walt Disney World, you wouldn't welcome a wheelchair as a support device!)

Fear of Falling

A very common fear for people with OA is that of falling down. There are two main reasons for this fear. First, you certainly don't want to hurt yourself. You may be afraid that if you fall, you'd really do a lot of damage. And second, you may be afraid that, once you fall, you won't be able to get back up!

What can you do? Try to be as careful as possible. Try to avoid hasty movements. Reorganize your environment to reduce the chances of tripping over anything. Beyond this, however, remind yourself that you can only do so much. You don't want to fall. But if it happens, it happens, and you'll deal with it then!

Fear of Others' Reactions

Are you afraid that other people will not accept you with osteoarthritis? Do you fear being shunned? You may fear rejection if you can't socialize the way you'd like to be able to. Others may feel that you can't keep up with them. But don't try, because pushing yourself can be a painful way to maintain a friendship.

Unfortunately, some people can be cold and unfeeling; they may have trouble dealing with the way you are because of your OA. If you're shaking your head saying "that doesn't apply to me," well, fine. You can move on to the next section. But some people do feel this way. If your friends care less about you, who needs those kinds of friends anyway? Other friends will accept you under any circumstances. Enjoy them. But since you can't change the way some people feel, try not to be as concerned with their reactions. Instead, be more attentive to your own needs and feelings.

Other fears in this category can be even more frightening. "What if my spouse leaves me? What if all my friends stay away from me?" Isolation can be a horrible thought. If it's not happening now, you may be afraid of it happening in the future. You may be afraid that none of your friends will remain "in your corner." To reduce the chances of such rejection, you may hesitate to make plans with friends or family. This will only add to your feeling of isolation.

Consider your thoughts, but be realistic. Remember that a change in a social relationship can occur for *any* reason, not just because of your condition! If you feel that your relationship is in jeopardy, see what you can do to help: "put all your cards on the table," discuss your problems, and even get counseling if it is needed. But you can only do so much. If that doesn't work, even though the outcome may upset you, at least you'll know you've tried.

Fear of Overdoing/Underdoing

You may not know how much you should do. You may be afraid of doing too much, but you may feel guilty about doing too little! How do you conquer this? Get advice from experts. You need professional advice in order to come up with the best "mix" of rest and exercise. This may become apparent only through trial and error. You can learn only through experience. One of the "advantages" of OA is that too much physical activity will signal you to slow down. Fortunately, rest can help painful joints feel better. Always remember to pace yourself. Change your level of activity gradually. Then tell yourself, as with so many other fears, that you're doing the best you can.

Fear of Employment Problems

You may be concerned about whether you'll be able to keep your job. You may want to work, but fear that you won't be able to. Your employer may be understanding at first, but you worry about how long this will continue. And, of course, you may be afraid of all the money problems that might result if you can't work. Because of all your financial obligations, you need money! If you can't work, this pressure is even greater. Medical bills have to be paid. You can't depend on insurance plans, since they don't always provide enough coverage. In addition, many insurance plans require that you pay the doctor first and then get reimbursed. Doctors' fees can be quite high, and if the money is not coming in . . .

Can you do much to change the nature of fear? Fortunately, many people with OA are able to keep working on their current job. But if you can't, you can evaluate your vocational skills and consider what jobs you'd be able to handle. And talk to people. Speak to others with OA who cannot work. See what they do. Maybe you'll get some ideas that will help you to conquer this fear.

Fear of Traveling

You may be reluctant to travel with OA. Why? You wouldn't know the doctors, what medical facilities were available, or who you could contact if you experienced a problem. Obviously, if you travel by car, this may not be much of a problem. But you want to be sure you can walk as much as you'd like and that your environment is conducive to getting around.

What can you do? By planning in advance, you should be able to answer these concerns. Ask your physician if he knows of any doctors or facilities in the area where you're planning to go. You might want to contact them in advance. If your physician has no contacts, either try to get some names on your own (try the local medical society or your local chapter of the Arthritis Foundation) or plan your vacation at a place where adequate medical services are available. Plan on not overdoing. Visiting five landmarks in one day is a bit much! (More about this in Chapter 21, "Traveling.")

Fear of Not Coping

You may feel that you're barely handling your OA. You may think that any new problem that comes along will be enough to push you over the edge. Fear of falling apart can easily lead to panic, an out-of-control kind of feeling that will make you fall apart. Get a hold of yourself. Pinpoint those particular things you're having difficulty with, and get help in dealing with them. Don't wait. Don't project a false sense of bravado that you can and must handle everything yourself. If you feel yourself near the edge, get someone to help you to steady yourself. Talk it over with someone. Once you share your feelings and fears with someone, you may see things a little more clearly. You may be able to deal with problems with greater strength, knowing that you're not alone. Once you're back in control, this fear will disappear.

A FEARLESS SUMMARY

Although many different fears have been discussed in this chapter, we have probably not covered all of the ones you have experienced. In addition, the coping suggestions offered certainly do not include all possible ways of dealing with fear. So what should you do?

You're working on recognizing your fears, right? For some of them, you're modifying your behavior. For others, you're modifying your thinking. Soon you will feel more in control. As this happens, you'll notice that your fears are beginning to diminish. That doesn't mean that they'll all go away. But as you work on them and feel more in control, they'll at least lessen in intensity. You'll feel better knowing that you can do something about some of them, and that you're capable of handling them.

8

Anger

Donna was fed up with joint pain. Practically anyone who went near her received an earful of comments you wouldn't want Mother to hear! Everyone was a victim of this verbal assault, from her doctor to her family. What made her even more angry was that she wanted to slam her fist down on her kitchen table, but she knew it would just make her pain worse. Donna was angry!

In general, people with any restrictive physical conditions may be angry. Because anger results in the build-up of physical energy that needs to be released, it is important to learn how to cope with anger.

WHAT IS ANGER?

When you have a desire or goal in mind, and something interferes with your achievement of it, a feeling of tension and hostility may result from the developing frustration. This is what we refer to as anger.

THREE TYPES OF ANGER

It can be helpful to discuss three different ways of experiencing anger. *Rage* is the expression of violent, uncontrolled anger. If Donna were feeling upset about her condition, and a "friend" told her that her joints would still be healthy if she had drunk three glasses of milk each day, you can imagine how angry she might be. Her anger might even lead her to say or do things that would certainly not enhance the prospects of a long, warm relationship with this person! Rage is probably the most intense anger you can experience. It is an outward expression of anger, one that results in a visible explosion. Rage can be a destructive release of the intense physical energy that builds up.

A second type of anger is *resentment*. This is the feeling of anger that is usually kept inside. What if Donna listened to her friend's well-meaning comments, smiled, and said nothing, but was seething inside? Resentment is a growing, smoldering feeling of anger directed toward a person or object. However, it is kept bottled up. It tends to sit uncomfortably within you, and can create even more physiological and psychological damage.

The third type of anger is *indignation*. Indignation is considered the more appropriate, positive type of anger. It is released in a more controlled way. If Donna had responded to the comments by stating that she appreciated her friend's concern, but would prefer no advice at this point or she might scream, this might have been a more appropriate response. Obviously, these three types of anger can occur in different ways. However, understanding the different ways of experiencing anger can help you to cope with it more effectively.

CAUSES OF ANGER

Obviously, there are lots of things that can make you angry. You may get angry if you keep breaking dishes because you can't hold them securely. You may get angry waiting for your doctor to see you. You may get angry if your doctor says you have arthritis, but doesn't mention which kind!

Insults from other people, aside from everyday frustrations, can cause anger. "If you didn't play so much tennis, your joints would still be working!" This is not the kind of comment that would make you feel friendly! If you feel that someone is taking advantage of you, or you feel forced to do something that you do not want to do, anger may result. If you do not have the ability or confidence to say "no" when friends ask for a favor, this can create feelings of anger, especially when combined with the fact that you may not feel well.

When thinking about the causes of anger, there may not be any specific reason you can point to. Or you might be able to list dozens of reasons. But understanding this is important, because you must be aware of the anger to help yourself deal with it. Unfortunately, resolving your anger won't eliminate the pain of OA. Nor should you say that you'll only stop being angry when OA is a thing of the past. Neither attitude will help you.

It is important to realize that anger exists uniquely in the mind of each angry individual. This anger is a direct result of your thoughts, rather than events. The event by itself does not make you angry. Rather, it leads to your *interpretation* of the event—the way you think or feel about it. That's what can make you angry. This is a very important point, one that will be discussed in much more detail a little bit later in the chapter, in the section "Dealing With Anger." Stay tuned. . . .

ANGER AND YOUR BODY

When you are angry, a number of physiological responses occur in your body. Breathing becomes more rapid, blood pressure increases (you may feel like your blood is "boiling"), and your heart may begin to pound. Your face may get "hot," and your muscles may become tense. You may feel stronger when angry. The more intense the anger is, the greater is this feeling of power. I'm sure you can remember a time when you were so angry that you felt you had superhuman strength.

Anger is a form of energy. The more physical energy that builds up in the body due to anger, the more necessary it becomes for you to release it. The energy cannot be destroyed, so if it is not released in some constructive manner, it will eventually come out in another, less desirable way. Imagine the energy from anger as a stick of dynamite about to explode. If you get rid of it, it will explode away from you. It may cause some damage, but it will not hurt you inside as much as if you swallowed the dynamite to keep others from being hurt. Obviously, the ideal solution is not to throw the stick of dynamite nor to swallow it, but (are you ready for this?) to try and defuse the dynamite! More about defusing soon.

Usually, extreme anger can pass quickly. If, however, the anger lasts for a long period of time, it can have physically damaging effects on the body. You've heard about some of the physical problems that can result from holding in anger: ulcers, hypertension, headaches. Anger can also make your OA worse. How? Anger causes you to "tense up," putting extra (and undesirable) pressure on your joints and muscles. It's just not good for your body.

When anger becomes extreme or turns into rage, you may feel like exploding. You may feel that unless you are able to punch, kick, or hit something to get rid of the anger in some way, you will lose control. Hopefully, this angry energy can be released without causing damage to another person, property, or yourself. If, when you finally calm down, you find that you have done something destructive, you may get angry at yourself all over again. Or you may experience another negative emotion, such as guilt.

ANGER AND YOUR MIND

Anger is usually experienced as an unpleasant feeling. However, this unpleasant feeling may exist along with a more pleasant feeling of power or strength. Frequently, the unpleasantness of anger is related to its consequences—knowing what you do when you are angry and not being happy about it. If you lose control when you're angry, you'll probably even be afraid of your anger, and of what you might do next time!

DIFFERENT REACTIONS TO ANGER

Marie, a 52-year-old teacher, was having a hard time with her husband. He was trying to show concern for his wife by not letting her do any housework. But, surprisingly, she *wanted* to clean the house because she believed she felt well enough to do it. His resistance was so persistent and he was so "saccharin sweet" that Marie felt it was too much. She wanted to be treated with respect, knowing that she was able to determine when she could be active. But her husband just wouldn't let up. She was running out of patience. Let's see how this situation might be experienced in different ways.

The "Ignore" Approach

Because you feel like you may completely lose control, or feel overwhelmed by the intensity of your anger, you may try to do whatever you can to avoid the experience. This could include pushing thoughts out of your mind, even when you realize you are getting angry. Marie might try to get involved in different activities while her husband cleans the house, and try to ignore the fact that he is being so condescending. Or she might try to agree with everything that he says. Although this might be upsetting, it might at least be temporarily effective in helping her to ignore the smothering. In the long run, however, you can see that this is not the best way to deal with anger.

The "Action" Approach

From another point of view, you might see anger as a necessary part of life, despite its unpleasantness. You know that there will be times when you're angry, whether you like it or not. You'll just have to deal with it as best you can.

In this case, Marie knows that she's not happy being angry, and that she should speak to her husband and try to get him to understand more about her emotional needs and how she'd like him to treat her. Hopefully, a better understanding can be reached, but at least Marie knows that she's doing something about her feelings.

The "Power" Approach

Maybe you enjoy the flow of energy and strength that comes from being angry. You may find that this is when you are best able to assert yourself to accomplish something. Here, Marie knows that if she is restrained once too often she will explode, and she loves the feeling of power that this anger gives her. She is almost looking forward to the chance to say, "Honey, if you treat me that way once more, I'll take this vacuum cleaner and . . . !" That would wipe the smile off hubby's face!

If you enjoy this feeling, it's possible that you may even provoke situations to make yourself angry! An example of this would be the professional football players or boxers who psyche themselves up before a confrontation with an opponent. For them, becoming as angry as possible is the best preparation for a successful performance.

Your own reaction to anger is unique. It may also change from time to time. There may be times when you accept anger and almost value it as a motivator to accomplish something. At other times you may attempt to push this anger away. Marie might enjoy expressing her anger. But if she doesn't want to cause problems with her husband, she might realize that it would be better to have a calm discussion with him than to shatter his eardrums with her explosion.

IS ANGER GOOD OR BAD?

How can anger possibly be good? Many people feel that nothing constructive can be gained from it. "Avoid anger at all costs," they say, "because nothing good comes from it. . . . Anger will get you into trouble, so don't let it happen." This is true, but only if you don't deal with the anger properly. Anger can be dangerous if it is kept inside. Remember that stick of dynamite? What an explosive example! If anger is released in destructive ways, it can cause problems in relationships (to say the least!). It can create physical problems as well, and can certainly aggravate your OA-related problems. Does this mean that anger can make your condition worse? Sure. What if you're so angry at somebody or something that you decide not to take proper care of yourself? For example, you don't get enough rest, or you don't do the prescribed amount of exercise. What if you're angry at someone who cares about you and normally helps around the house? That person, if upset by your anger, may be less willing to help you. This may, in turn, make you feel even worse. So if you want your anger to be good instead of bad, try to turn it into something that can be helpful rather than harmful to you.

Anger can be constructive. It can mobilize your efforts and make you stronger to deal with an anger-provoking situation. Believe it or not, you might even handle a situation more successfully when you're angry than when you're not! Anger can give you a feeling of power or strength, of confidence or assertiveness. But don't misunderstand me. I'm not saying that you should slam your finger with a hammer or tell someone to punch you in order to get yourself angry enough to solve all of your problems! What I am saying is that anger can be positive, and it can help you to solve problems. Anger has two main benefits. First, it is an indicator that something is wrong. Something must be creating this feeling of anger—something that needs attention. Second, anger can motivate you to deal more actively with life's problems. You can become so emotionally charged that it will have a positive effect on your life.

In order for anger to be helpful, there are some very important things to keep in mind. First, don't let yourself become overwhelmed by anger. Once that happens it is much harder to do what you have to do. Second, don't be afraid of your anger. If you do fear it, you probably won't be able to release it properly. More than likely, it will come out in unhealthy ways, or you'll bottle it up inside. Third, be sure that the way you handle your anger is socially acceptable. Marie might get a kick out of knocking out her husband's teeth, but would the dentist (or the police) approve? Try to be flexible enough to recognize an appropriate way of releasing your anger.

DEALING WITH ANGER

You've already begun to realize that anger can be constructive. Hopefully, the information you've read so far has been encouraging. But what else can actually be done to handle anger?

Because anger is such a complex emotion, and because so many things can lead to feelings of anger, there are no simple answers. Sorry about that! Does that mean that there is nothing that anybody can do about anger? No. Some things can be done to reduce the feelings of anger and allow them to be handled more efficiently, comfortably, and safely.

Step One—Admit That You're Angry

The first step in dealing with anger is to recognize that you're angry. As simple as this may sound, many people cannot even admit when they are angry. They may try to deny it or to rationalize their feelings or behaviors using other explanations. Do you feel that being angry is a sign of weakness? If so, since you don't want to feel weak, you may not even admit that you're angry. You may feel that there is no appropriate reason to be angry and that you're acting in a childish way. But as with anything else, in order to try to change something, you've got to first admit that it exists.

How can you tell that you're angry if you're not sure? (Yes, there are some people who are not sure.) If you feel very tense (jumping at the sound of the telephone), or if you find yourself reacting impulsively (slamming down the phone when you get a wrong number and storming out of the house) or with hostility (cursing at your neighbor for leaving a smidgeon of garbage on your lawn), chances are that you're angry. Until you recognize that you are angry, you cannot do anything constructive about it.

Step Two—Identify the Source of Your Anger

The second step in dealing with anger is trying to identify its source. Where does it come from? What is contributing to it? What events have led to these feelings of anger? Why do you want to break all the furniture? For one thing, your condition may lead to anger. You may be angry with yourself for neglecting your condition. You may feel anger toward your physician, whether justified or not. You may be angry because you have to take so much pain medication. You may be angry because of the things you can no longer do.

In some cases, the events leading to anger may be quite obvious. In other cases, however, the source of anger may be vague and unclear. It may be hard to pinpoint what is causing it. At such times, you should try to probe even more deeply to come up with possible causes of your anger.

Of course, much of this anger is irrational. But like other emotional reactions, it must be worked through. It cannot just be pushed away. Simply telling yourself not to be angry is not enough. You must learn to channel your anger more effectively.

Step Three—Identify the Reason for Your Anger

It is now necessary to explain to yourself why you are angry. Why is this step important? Mainly, to decide whether the anger that you are feeling is realistic. Analyze your reasons for being angry. If you recognize that your reasons are not realistic, this alone can help you to deal with these feelings of anger. If, on the other hand, you can objectively say that your feelings of anger are realistic, then the next step is to decide how you are going to deal with them properly.

How do you deal with them properly? You have already begun! By working through the first three steps, you have received information that will be very helpful in your efforts to deal with your anger.

THOUGHTS CAN MAKE YOU ANGRY

In the past, it was mistakenly believed that there were only two possible ways to deal with anger: to keep it inside or to let it out.

But what about a third possibility? Remember before when we talked about defusing that stick of dynamite? Our anger is a result of the way we think! In our minds, we are actually interpreting those events that lead to anger. If we can change the way we interpret events, and reorganize our thinking patterns, is it possible to stop creating the anger that we feel? Of course! We can learn to control our thoughts *before* they make us angry, regardless of what the events were. Ask yourself this question: Would something that makes you angry make everybody angry? No. You are angry because of the way you think about or interpret the event. Other people aren't angry because they did not interpret the event in a way that would make them so. Let's say, for example, that you'd made a doctor's appointment. Ten minutes before you were ready to leave, the receptionist called to cancel, saying she'd reschedule the appointment at another time. You might be furious, because you felt you should have received more notice, and because you really wanted to see the doctor. How aggravating!! But others might not interpret it that way, and might not get the least bit angry. So if we can learn to interpret events in a more positive, constructive, and calm manner, we can reduce feelings of anger. We wouldn't have to decide whether we wanted to let anger out or keep it inside because, by controlling our thoughts, anger would not even exist most of the time.

You've already completed one of the first steps in reorganizing your thoughts to prevent anger. You've learned that anger can be good and constructive. It can help you to solve problems, and you don't have to be afraid of it. Just becoming aware of its positive elements can help you to be less afraid of anger. This can help you deal with the thoughts that may make you angry.

Good Angry Thoughts Versus Bad Angry Thoughts

Writing down what you think is making you angry can be very helpful. Good angry thoughts can move you to positive, constructive action. You might want to plan your strategies for resolving the problem. On the other hand, many of your thoughts may include so much anger and be so destructive that you feel like banging your head against the wall. Be honest when writing down your thoughts, regardless of how violent or profane they may be. Such rich, colorful language can be helpful in getting your feelings out. This will ultimately help you to control your anger. Try to look at these thoughts more objectively, the way someone else might look at them. Attempt to bring them down to a more manageable level.

Mental Movies

An interesting technique that can be helpful in controlling anger is imagery, or "watching movies in your mind." When you become angry, you frequently have all kinds of pictures in your head of what is making you angry and what you'd like to do to deal with it. These movies can be very beneficial.

For example, imagine that you are very, very tired. Your friend calls to tell you that her car has broken down. Could you please pick up her dry cleaning? When you tell her that your joints are too sore to pick up lint, much less dry cleaning, she says something about how she can never depend on you for anything. This is a friend? You are furious. At that moment, imagine all the abusive things that you would like to say to her, and imagine the shocked expression on her face. If you ask her to hold on for a moment, close your eyes, and imagine this as if you were actually doing it, you'll probably be able to complete the phone call without destroying a friendship. You may even smile or laugh as you think about the scenes that are playing through your mind. More about imagery in Chapter 14, "Pain."

Ruth was quite fed up with her husband, Messy Max. Whenever she asked for his help with normal household chores, his answers were fresh and abusive. Just before she was about to give him a haircut with a meat cleaver, she remembered the mental movie technique. She imagined herself strangling him—his eyeballs popping out and gurgling sounds coming from this throat. This helped to get rid of the intense, angry feelings that were making her crazy, and allowed her to deal with Max more constructively. (No, she's not in jail.)

The Big, Red Stop Sign

Another technique that can help you to control anger is referred to as "thought stopping." Remember: It is the thoughts in your mind that are making you angry. These are the thoughts you have when interpreting an event. When you find that angry thoughts have come into your head, picture a big, red stop sign. Seeing that word in your mind will serve as a momentary distraction. Then concentrate on something you enjoy, whether it is a peaceful, relaxing scene, a type of food that you like to eat, an activity that you enjoy, or a movie or television program. Whatever you choose, you will divert your thinking, and have a better chance of dissipating your anger. You could also participate in a pleasant distracting activity, such as reading a book, taking a walk, or calling a friend, which will also help you to feel less angry.

Change Your Requirements

People often get angry when they want certain things to occur in particular ways. When your specific requirements are not met, you may feel angry. Trying to modify your requirements can help you to cope with anger.

Let's say that you're not feeling well and you decide to call your doctor. The answering service tells you that he is not in the office and that you should get a return call within a half-hour. After forty-five minutes, when he still has not returned your call, you are fuming. Why? Because your requirement of a response within thirty minutes has not been met. Revise your requirement. Tell yourself that you would have liked a call within thirty minutes, but your doctor may be tied up on another case, in transit, or unable to get to a phone. You'll be satisfied if you get a call at his earliest convenience. By modifying the requirement, you can feel less angry.

Another way to benefit from this technique is to write down those thoughts indicating what your requirements are. Then try to write down new, more flexible desires. This will make you feel better.

PUT YOURSELF IN THEIR SHOES

One of the best ways of dealing with anger toward somebody else is to try to understand exactly what that person is feeling, what the person wants, and why the person is saying what he or she is saying. This will make you more aware of why someone else is behaving or talking the way he or she is, and you will be better able to deal with it constructively. You will also better understand how the other person feels when he or she is the target of your abusive release of anger.

LET IT OUT LESS EXPLOSIVELY

We have discussed a number of ways to control your thinking and improve your ability to interpret events in ways that will not allow anger to develop. But what if this doesn't always work? What if there are times when you remain as angry as you were before? What can be done to deal with anger constructively when it already exists?

Talk, Don't Bite

Obviously, it is much more desirable to have a constructive discussion over an issue than an angry exchange of heated words, which accomplishes nothing. In most cases, anger arises from a conflict or problem with another person. Therefore, it is frequently helpful to improve your ability to get your point across effectively. You are trying to negotiate a better resolution to a problem that may exist between you and somebody else. Heated arguments and "fighting fire with fire" are not the answer. Instead, you want to fight the fire by dousing it, reducing the heatedness of the argument. Try complimenting the person. Or look for the positive things in what that person is saying to you, even if you're angry. This works in two ways. One, it will probably surprise the person. Two, you'll be focusing on words or thoughts that are more constructive, rather than letting yourself get angry because of what's being said. You can calmly restate your feelings.

Get Involved in an Activity

In general, one of the best outlets for releasing angry energy is activity. Because of OA, though, this outlet may not be as available as you'd like. Interestingly, it has been found that physical energy from anger can be released by watching things. For example, by watching a sporting event, you aren't releasing energy through participation in the sport, but you may still be able to "get into it" and reduce your anger that way. Or try watching a particularly violent or emotionally draining movie. You can become so totally absorbed that the energy building up from anger is released through worry, fear, or excitement.

A movie or book that allows you to identify with the characters, or where the characters allow release of anger, can be beneficial as well. A common and very effective outlet for anger, especially among children, is crying. I'm sure you've heard of the therapeutic effects of a good cry. However, this technique is not for everyone. People who can be more open in expressing their emotions may be better able to benefit from this outlet.

Some people like to count to ten when angry. This can distract you from what is making you angry, giving you a chance to calm down and think about it more constructively. Try counting to a thousand, if necessary!

LET US REVIEW

It is very important to remember that events alone do not make you angry. It is your thoughts, your interpretations of these events, that lead to anger. Even if something really terrible happens, it is the meaning that you give to this particular event that makes you angry. It is the way you think about this horrible event that creates your anger. Since your thinking makes you angry, you are responsible for feeling this way. Therefore, you can be just as responsible for changing your thinking to help yourself cope with anger, or at least reducing it to a more manageable level.

The best way to handle anger is probably to be in control enough, so that it doesn't build up in the first place. But if it does, remember that if anger is channeled and used constructively, it does have its benefits. Uncontrolled anger can be an unpleasant, negative, destructive emotion. Your efforts are best spent trying to figure out how to reorganize your thinking so that it doesn't get out of hand.

9
Guilt

Have you ever felt guilty? Many individuals with OA say that they have. Guilt is a very unpleasant emotion. Take the case of Rosie. She was very unhappy because she couldn't knit sweaters for her grandchildren anymore. She felt she wasn't being the kind of grandmother she wanted to be. Why not? Well, because she just couldn't participate in enough activities with her kids. So having OA made her feel guilty that she was being a bad grandmother. Hard to cope? You bet! Let's take a look at what leads to guilty feelings.

THE TWO COMPONENTS OF GUILT

Feelings of guilt usually have two components. The first of these is the "wrongdoing"; you feel that you have either done something wrong or haven't done something that you should have done. The second component is the "self-blame"; you blame yourself for doing this wrong thing, and feel that you are "bad" because of it. That's the culprit! It is the concept of "badness" that creates the guilty feeling. If you *feel* bad about doing something wrong, this is normal and understandable. But when you start telling yourself that you *are* bad, guilt follows. What if other people tell you that the way you feel is O.K.? This may not help. Your feeling of guilt may have nothing to do with what others tells you or what they think. Even if they disagree with you, these are still your feelings. Remember: Your guilt comes from feeling that you are a bad person, rather than from feeling bad about what you have done. Is it fitting to label yourself as a bad person or blame yourself because you've done something wrong? Even if you have done something wrong, it's better to label that particular behavior as bad, rather than yourself.

Is the behavior that you are blaming yourself for really that terrible or wrong? Does it justify the feeling of badness that leads to guilt? In Rosie's case, then, she felt guilty because of her OA. Does that make sense? Did she make it happen? Of course not. Rosie might have felt better, therefore, if she had emphasized the quality of time spent with her children, rather than the gifts she made for them.

WHAT IS VERSUS WHAT OUGHT TO BE

Guilt feelings about the inability to handle household chores are very common for women with OA. On the other hand, men tend to feel more guilty about the inability to fulfill their job responsibilities the way they feel they should. How about Ralph, a 52-year-old car salesman. He felt guilty because he was not able to work as efficiently at his job as he used to. He therefore earned less money—not enough to provide all of the luxuries he and his family would have enjoyed. Feeling pressured, Ralph tried to work harder to earn more money, which in turn made him feel worse physically. This created the guilty feelings. He felt less capable of being the breadwinner in the family, and believed he was therefore a bad father and husband. How can you cope with these feelings?

Do you see a difference between the way you are doing something and the way you think you should be doing it? If so, you may really feel guilty! How do you work this out? Major union/management problems would be easier to solve! Can you work harder or do more? If you can, then do it. If not, try examining your day-to-day goals for working and living. Check to see if these goals are practical, considering what you can and cannot do because of your OA. Try to take more pride in what you can do. Although most people hate hearing, "Things could be worse," this phrase is quite true. You might not be able to do anything at all. If you concentrate on the things you can do and place less emphasis on what you can't do, your feelings of guilt will diminish. You'll feel a lot better. Changing the emphasis in your thinking will also help you to lessen the gap between what is and what ought to be. This is what led to these guilty feelings in the first place.

Does this approach work only for working men? No. It applies to anyone who feels guilty about falling short of expectations and desires. Thelma was upset because she was unable to prepare cakes for the PTA bake sale the way she used to. She felt embarrassed and guilty, as if she single-handedly were going to cost the school money! How might Thelma have coped with these guilty feelings? It might have been beneficial for Thelma to speak to school officials and explain how OA was affecting her, asking if there were other ways that she might be able to help. In this way, the feelings of guilt related to having OA would have decreased.

TALK IT OVER

It is very important to discuss how you feel about your condition with others who may be affected by it. It is helpful to talk over feelings with the important people in your life, to share concerns, and to try to figure out solutions to problems. Jane, a 58-year-old woman who had been married for over thirty years, enjoyed going square dancing with her husband twice each week. (No squares, these two!) In addition, she and her husband would participate in other social activities with friends at least one or two other evenings each week. Now because of the pain she was experiencing from OA, she had to restrict her activities. She just couldn't go out as frequently. She couldn't even do-si-do her partner! Sometimes, she wouldn't want to go out even once during an entire week. Not only did she feel unhappy about her condition, but she felt extremely guilty about holding her husband back. She felt that he couldn't have a good time because of her. It would have been helpful for Jane to discuss alternatives with her husband. If she had arrived at a solution with her husband's cooperation, she could have effectively reduced guilt feelings and improved the marriage.

THOUGHTS CAN HURT, TOO

So far, we have discussed how doing the wrong thing can lead to guilt. But it's not only "behavioral mistakes" that can lead to guilty feelings. Thoughts can also become upsetting enough to lead to guilt.

Sometimes, you may feel guilty without having done anything wrong. You may merely think of things that cause guilt. Penny, a 51-year-old mother of three, was feeling terribly guilty. Why? Her 53-year-old husband was spending many hours doing things for the kids that she felt she should be doing. Heavens, he was even helping with the housework! Penny knew that her condition meant that she couldn't do what she used to, but she felt bad because her husband had to do so much. She was afraid that he would eventually start complaining. Should Penny have blamed herself and felt guilty because of her condition—something she could not control? Since she hadn't really done anything wrong, Penny would have felt better if she had modified her thinking.

In order to successfully cope with guilt, you must first focus on what led to the guilty feelings. Have you actually done something wrong? Have you really neglected something you shouldn't have? You may feel guilty about your thoughts or desires, rather than specific actions or behaviors. Recognize that if you haven't done anything to lead to guilt, then you should identify those thoughts that are making you feel like a bad person. Change them. If you can learn to talk to yourself in a positive way, looking at your thoughts objectively and constructively, guilt can be reduced.

Frequently, as in Penny's case, feeling guilty is related to seeing yourself as responsible for others' actions or behaviors. The more responsible you feel, the more guilt you may feel, especially if you cannot fulfill your responsibility. Frequently, just asking the question "why?" will point out that this thinking is unrealistic and will help to reduce guilt. This is another reason why discussions with the people closest to you are helpful. They may explain why taking the responsibility for someone else is inappropriate. Be sure to place feelings of responsibility in proper perspective. There is a limit to how responsible you should feel for others' actions or feelings. Nor are you responsible for having OA or for any restrictions this may place on you. Penny should have recognized that nobody was forcing her husband to take over her household responsibilities. He chose this course of action. Penny would have experienced less guilt if she hadn't felt responsible for her husband's choice. Realize that when individuals are not forced to take part in an activity, they participate out of choice and desire. The same holds true for this book. You are reading it out of choice and desire, aren't you?

"SHOULD" THOUGHTS

Among the most common causes of guilt are thoughts containing the word "should." "Should" is a dirty word! Examples of such thoughts are: "I should have been able to finish that job today," "We should have that party; all our friends have entertained us this year," and "You should have let me do the dishes." These "should" thoughts imply that you must be just about perfect and on top of everything. When there is a difference between what you feel should occur and what actually does occur, guilt can result. You will become upset whenever you fall short of your "should." Should thoughts lead to guilt simply because they are not sensible, realistic, or justifiable? Should you blame yourself because you have chosen goals that you may not be able to fulfill?

Now that I've explained what you *shouldn't* do, what exactly should you do? In order to feel better and reduce feelings of guilt, it is helpful to reword your thoughts to eliminate "should" thoughts. Try to use less demanding words. Say, "It would be nice if I could finish that job today, but I can't," rather than, "I should finish that job today." If your physical condition is restricting your activities, you'll feel much more guilty when "should" thoughts remind you of unfulfilled obligations. If you have trouble changing the wording of your "should" thoughts, try asking yourself, "Why should I...?" or "Who says I should...?" or "Where is it written that I should...?" This may help you decide whether you are setting up impossible requirements for yourself. It can also help reduce your feelings of guilt.

Let's say, for example, that you are thinking of giving a party because all your friends have invited you to get-togethers. Ask yourself why you should. Is it because the "Party Rulebook" tells you so? If you don't have a party, will your friendship license be revoked? If you don't have a party, won't your friends (some friends!) invite you to their homes anymore? As you think about the realistic answers to these questions, it will be easier to realize that you don't have to have a party. Although giving a party would be nice, it is more acceptable to think of other ways of reciprocating if, physically, you are unable to have a party.

THE CONSEQUENCES OF GUILT

So far, we've been discussing what leads to guilt, how you may feel, and how you can try to adjust your thoughts and behaviors to feel better. But what happens if you have not yet been successful in eliminating guilt? People who feel guilty frequently act in negative ways to hide from these feelings. There may be a tendency to indulge in "escape" behaviors, such as drinking or excessive sleeping, that do not deal with problems head-on but, instead, attempt to push them away.

Joe, a 67-year-old bookkeeper, felt guilty because he had stopped making plans with his friends. He did this because he could no longer hold playing cards in his hands, and felt that his friends would no longer be interested in getting together with him. As a result, he did begin to lose friends, and his guilt became more and more difficult to bear. He began drinking each day, in an attempt to "escape" and forget his misery. This behavior did not help the situation. In fact, it was downright dangerous. Not only did it compound the problem, but there was the added danger of mixing alcohol and medication. Now Joe had something else to feel guilty about: his escape behavior. This could increase his feeling of badness, leading to even more guilt and creating a vicious circle.

The first step toward improvement is to look past the escape behavior and identify whatever is causing the guilt. Consider what can be done to rectify the problem causing the guilt. At the same time, try to eliminate any escape behavior, recognizing that it is only a cop-out. It is possible, however, for there to be no clear-cut solution to the events or feelings creating guilt. If, for example, Joe's physical condition kept him from holding playing cards, aren't there devices that could do this for him? Or does he really believe that his friends would only want to see him if he were a card player? That would be ridiculous. Don't give up because no complete solution exists. Look for partial solutions that can still help to reduce guilt by reminding you that you are trying to improve the situation. Joe's OA won't go away, but he can at least try to reduce his reluctance to get together with friends. There must be other things they can do!

OTHER SUGGESTIONS

We've talked a lot about how thoughts and behaviors can cause guilt. But what if you just feel guilty and can't remember what you were thinking or doing to make you feel that way? How can you start using all these great thought-changing ideas if you don't remember what thoughts you want to change? Good question! In order to identify those "target" thoughts or behaviors, you might want to keep a brief written log of feelings or activities that may have caused your guilt. Once you have written these things down, you can then begin figuring out how to change them, improve your outlook, and reduce your guilt.

Betty, age 75, had been feeling increasingly guilty but didn't really know why. By keeping a log, she noticed that she hadn't been calling her children as often, because her fingers hurt so much she didn't want to dial the phone. The log helped her realize that she did want to call them more, so she decided to buy a new Touch-Tone pushbutton phone with memory. Now she could call, even if she had to press the buttons with her nose! As she resolved the problem, her guilt disappeared.

What about those negative thoughts that lead to guilt? It can be very helpful to try to turn these thoughts around, making them more positive and guilt-free. For example, let's say that you feel guilty because you believe you are a bad husband or wife. Ask yourself if you have ever done anything that a good spouse might do. Just about every person can come up with something. This starts the process of eliminating your "bad spouse blues." The idea is to turn your mind's negative thoughts into reasonable, positive ones. This way, the feeling of guilt will not take a stranglehold!

A FINAL GUILTY THOUGHT

Guilt is a very destructive emotion—one that can certainly interfere with your success in coping with osteoarthritis. By becoming aware of how guilt develops, you will have a much better chance of effectively employing coping strategies to reduce guilt and its negative effects.

10

Stress

What is stress? Stress is a response that occurs in your body. It helps you mobilize your strength to deal with different things happening in your life. Many things occur each day that require you to adapt. These are the "stressors." All the changes that occur in your body when something (the stressor) provokes you are known as the "stress response."

With osteoarthritis, you may experience stress for many reasons. For example, pain alone can cause stress. Your concern about whether your disease will get worse can cause stress. Worries about joint replacement surgery can be stressful. Problems with medication are also stressors. Any one of these—and more—can provoke the stress response.

IS STRESS GOOD OR BAD?

A certain amount of stress is normal and necessary. Stress helps you to "get your act together," and prepares you to handle your life in the best possible way. Now you're probably thinking, "So why do I always hear people talking about how stress can be harmful?" When people talk about the harmful effects of stress, they are referring to situations in which there is *too much* stress. If stress is left unchecked, it can eat away at you and drain all of your energy.

Reasonable amounts of stress can be handled. In fact, they can even be helpful. This chapter, however, is concerned with harmful stress—the kind that can hurt if not controlled. The word "stress" is used very frequently these days. It describes those things that create nervousness, anxiety, tension, anger, or an upset feeling. Although these are all possible reactions to stress, they are not synonymous. In other words, they result from the stress response.

Frances, a 55-year-old housewife, was under pressure. Her husband was bringing his boss home for dinner. In an attempt to minimize the pain in her joints, she carefully paced herself as she prepared the meal so she wouldn't have to stop altogether. The stress she felt was tolerable—that is, until the phone rang. Her husband called, telling her that due to an emergency business meeting that evening, they'd be arriving two hours early! Frances's stress was no longer tolerable!

WHO FEELS STRESS?

Everyone experiences stress. Nobody escapes it. But since stress can be positive or negative, learning how to respond positively will lead to more stable emotional and physical states. If you have a hard time responding to stress, this won't be easy. Some people are more vulnerable to negative stress responses than others. Are you?

THE STRESS RESPONSE

Every person has a unique way of dealing with stress. Stress management (effectively managing the way you respond to stress) is within your reach. The way you cope depends on a number of things—your upbringing, your self-esteem, your beliefs about yourself and the world, what you say to yourself, and how you guide yourself in your thoughts and actions. The degree to which you feel in control of your life plays a role in your reaction to stress. The way you feel physically and emotionally, and the way you get along with people, are also a part of it. To sum it up, everyone's method of dealing with stress is unique, depending upon a complex combination of thoughts and behaviors.

Stressor + Interpretation = Stress Response

The way in which you are affected by stress depends on the "chemistry" between two factors. The first factor is the stressor, or the outside pressures. What is going on around you that is creating the reaction? The second factor is what is within you, or how you interpret things. It is the interaction of the stimulus and your own internal reaction that determines the way in which you're affected by stress. (Sound familiar? Yes, it's the same "formula" that can be applied to anger, depression, and all the other emotions.) This equation has important implications for coping with stress, if you realize that it isn't just the environment that causes you stress, but also the way you interpret the stressor. Some stressors in the environment would produce stress in anybody. What would happen, for example, if somebody pointed a knife at your throat? Calm acceptance or a stress response? Get the point? It's important to learn how to reduce the number of stressors that negatively affect you, and to improve your reaction to those you can't avoid.

Body Versus Mind

How do you respond to stress? Like your response to anger or other mobilizing emotions, there are two main ways: physically and cognitively. A cognitive response includes the way you think and feel. Most people react to stress in both ways, although it is possible for you to respond in only one way.

What happens physically? When you experience a stressful situation, the circulatory system speeds up. Blood is pushed rapidly toward different parts of the body, particularly those parts necessary to protect you. Because the blood supply is diverted toward these essential parts, the supply to the digestive system is usually reduced. As a result, the digestive process slows down, making it work less efficiently.

Chronic or prolonged stress puts a severe strain on your body. When your body is strong, it can fight off most foreign invaders, bacteria, and germs. As a result, many diseases can be avoided. But prolonged stress puts such a strain on your body that your defense mechanisms may break down. This, in turn, makes your body more vulnerable to the very problems you'd like to avoid!

Have you heard of the "fight or flight" syndrome? Animals do this when they feel threatened. The animal prepares either to fight or run away, a purely physical response. You will not see an animal standing there, scratching his head and thinking about what should be done! But humans have the unique ability to think and reason! Lucky us! So we include cognitive responses in our repertoire. (By the way, researchers feel that this is one of the main reasons why human beings are so susceptible to stress-related physical illness. By thinking, instead of acting, we are not dealing with stress as effectively as we might.)

When does stress lead to physical problems? When you can't respond to stress in a way that eliminates it, the stress continues unabated. The inability to do something about it may cause even more stress, creating a vicious cycle. This can take its toll on your body.

You may be vulnerable to stress in your own unique way. Certain parts of your body may tend to be more vulnerable to the effects of stressors. For example, have you ever felt extreme intestinal discomfort and automatically clutched your stomach because of stress? Or have you ever endured a painful headache? Stress may have even exacerbated your OA, or played a role in another illness or condition that you've suffered.

What happens if you respond to stress physically? You may tremble or perspire. Your face may flush. You may feel a surge of adrenaline flowing through your body. Your mouth may become dry or you may feel nauseated. Your breathing may become more rapid and shallow. Your heart may begin to pound. Your muscles may become tight, creating headaches, cramps, or other painful reactions. Sounds lovely, doesn't it?

Your cognitive or emotional response to stress may not be as visible. You may not be able to concentrate as well. Your attention span may be reduced. You may have trouble learning something new. You may be afraid to do things. You may withdraw or feel nervous. You may lose confidence in yourself. You'll become aware of the unpleasant physical responses resulting from stress, and this may make you feel even more stressed. For example, if you feel stress and respond with shallow, rapid breathing or heart palpitations, your awareness of these physical responses may lead to feelings of panic and create even more stress.

THREE REACTIONS TO STRESS

When a stressful stimulus occurs, you will most likely react in one of three ways. You might react immediately and impulsively without giving enough thought to a better response. You might not react at all, and either try to ride it out or become so frozen that you are unable to respond. Finally, you might react to stressors in a well-planned, organized, and effective manner. If so, you might not even need this chapter! But if not, read on!

HOW TO DEAL WITH STRESS

Remember: Stress can be managed and controlled, but it cannot be eliminated. Stress will always exist. You can learn how to deal with different amounts of stress, but you'll never be able to make it go away. For a person with OA, it is especially important that stress be controlled. Why? Although stress by itself does not cause OA, it can certainly play a role in increasing your OA pain.

Let's begin by mentioning the wrong ways of responding to stress. These are the ways that won't help you: smoking, getting drunk, using drugs, overeating, and overactivity. Not only will these activities distract you and delay the effects of stress, but they can also hurt you.

So what should you do? Try to learn new, more appropriate ways of dealing with stress than the methods you've been using.

Relaxation Procedures

The best way to start controlling stress is by using relaxation procedures. Try the "quick release" method discussed in the introductory chapter of this section. Other successful methods of relaxation include meditation, self-hypnosis, imagery, and even a warm shower! Deep breathing alone can help to eliminate tension from the body, slow down the heart, and create a greater sense of well-being. Learning to relax can be helpful in reducing the amount of stress you are experiencing. It will give your body a chance to rest and recuperate as well. When your body is stronger, you'll be able to deal more effectively with the ravages of stress (or of life)! Relaxation will also help you to sleep better. Wouldn't that be nice?

Pinpointing Stressors

In order to learn how to cope with stress successfully, you must first identify your stressors. What, specifically, is causing you to feel stress? Maybe you're having trouble dealing with the never-ending pain. Maybe you're concerned about medication. Maybe you fear surgery. Maybe you're just having a hard time with other symptoms of osteoarthritis. These are all possible OA-related stressors, and, of course, there are plenty more.

What if you're not sure what's causing the stress? How can you figure out what it is? One way is to keep a record of your activities and experiences, using numerical ratings such as those in the SUD scale. SUD stands for Subjective Units of Disturbance. How does it work? Ratings on this scale range from 0 to 100, depending on the amount of stress you're experiencing. Use 100 to represent the most extreme and disturbing stress, and 0 to represent no stress (total and complete relaxation). Then rate your activities and experiences on the SUD scale. The ones with the higher SUD numbers are the ones causing you the most stress. For example, loud, blasting music from a teenager's radio might be rated a whopping 85!

Identifying Stress Reactions

Once you have begun identifying your stressors, you must then become completely aware of your responses to them. Are they more physiological or psychological? What parts of your body seem to be the most vulnerable? What kind of reaction does your body show? Does your attention span suffer? Do you start losing confidence or feel like you're slipping? As you become more aware of these changes, you will develop a more complete picture of your unique stress response. You'll be able to recognize the stressors that affect you and how you react to them. You'll then be better able to decide whether you should modify your behavior in response to the stressor.

What's the next step? Once you have recognized which stressors are negative, try to determine whether you can eliminate them. If you can, start figuring out how to do it. Removing the source of stress is an obvious and logical way to manage stress. Develop a plan of attack. This might include a number of alternative strategies, all designed to remove or minimize the impact of the stressor. Taking a sledgehammer to that radio might be great, but only if you can lift the hammer!

But what happens if you can't eliminate the source of your stress? You'll then have to work on your thoughts and responses in order to manage stress. In such cases, you won't be able to change the stressor, but you will be able to change the way you react. You might want to use some of the suggestions discussed in Chapters 6 and 8. The use of systematic desensitization, which was discussed in Chapter 7, also can be beneficial. Many techniques for changing your thinking have already been presented in previous chapters.

Relieving Physical Stress

Certain physical activities can be great for stress control. For example, some people can relieve tension or stress by driving. As long as the driver continues to observe safety rules, driving can be very relaxing.

Another important way of dealing with stress is by exercising. As you'll read later, exercise is not only important in helping you deal with stress, it is one of the most essential components of your treatment program for OA. Regardless of how OA is affecting you, there are still exercises you can do to help control stress. Virtually any type of exercise can be effective. Anything that gets the body moving, gets the heart pumping faster, and releases tension is ideal.

Hobbies or other leisure activities can be very helpful. They can divert your attention from the stressful situation, directing it toward something more enjoyable. These activities will also help you feel productive. A lack of productivity may be one of the stressors giving you problems in the first place!

Another technique for dealing with stress is sleep. Some people have difficulty sleeping when experiencing high levels of stress. However, you may not be one of those people and might be able to take naps to reduce stress.

IN CONCLUSION

What are your goals? If stress is interfering with your achievement of these goals, then your stress response is negative. If you learn how to control stress, then you can realize your goals and better cope with osteoarthritis.

11

Other Emotions

The emotions we've covered so far in this section are not the only ones, of course. Worry, for example, is a basic emotion. What might you worry about? Have you got a month to discuss all the possibilities? You've probably worried about the future, what your life will be like, whether you should have a joint replaced, how life will change because of osteoarthritis, among countless other things. What other emotions enter into the picture? This chapter will discuss four other emotions common for people with OA: boredom, envy, loneliness, and upset.

ARE YOU BORED?

Hopefully, by this time, you are not so bored that you have stopped reading! As long as you aren't bored, let's talk a little about boredom. What an empty feeling! It's one of the worst feelings anyone can experience. It has been said that more problems and serious tragedies come from being bored than from any other single condition.

Why are you bored? There may be no meaningful activity going on, no stimulation or excitement. Your life may seem to be going nowhere. Nothing is challenging you, and there's no incentive to do anything. Because you weren't born bored, you must have learned how to be bored. You weren't always bored, and even now you are not always bored. There are still certain things that hold your attention from time to time. Right?

Is Osteoarthritis Boring?

I bet you never thought of osteoarthritis as boring. But it can be, primarily because of the restrictions that your condition may impose on you. Some activities that provided enjoyment for you in the past may now be out of reach.

Olive hated the fact that her condition prevented her from knitting. She was tired of music, and she didn't want to read. Was Olive bored? Definitely! But did she have to be bored? No! Her family and friends suggested that she try new activities, and Olive soon was able to feel less bored.

So what should you do? Don't let your condition cause you to give up living. Distinguish between what you can do and what you can't. If you do have to curtail any activities because of osteoarthritis, you'll do so. If you have to drop an activity, you'll drop it. But you don't have to eliminate all activitites from your life simply because you feel you won't complete them.

"Unboring" Yourself

What can you do about it? The first step is to analyze why you are bored. What is causing the boredom? Obviously, figuring this out will help you determine how you can improve things. Then you'll want to see what you can do to add some interest to your life. But don't feel that you must push yourself to enjoy something. Forcing yourself to be amused rarely works. You may find that activities you used to enjoy have become artificial and uninteresting. You may no longer get any pleasure from them. That doesn't mean, however, that you should give up and not try to do something. You'll want to engage in some new activities to make your life more interesting. Don't limit yourself to those things that used to interest you. Preferences change. Try things that never interested you before, because maybe now they will spark new interest in you.

Learn Something New!

One of the most effective weapons against boredom is learning. The mind is like a sponge, constantly soaking up more information and knowledge. Select a potentially interesting topic you don't know much about. Try to learn something about it. You may want to begin by going to the library and reading some books on the topic. Maybe you'd like to enroll in an adult education course. Often, boredom quickly disappears once you are involved in something new.

You can also become bored if your social life is not the greatest. What can you do about this? Once again, try to learn something, especially by taking courses of some kind. Aside from the mental stimulation you'll get from such activities, you may also meet interesting and challenging people. Increasing your circle of friends is a good way to fight boredom.

Anticipation!

One of the best ways to fight boredom is to always give yourself something to look forward to. It doesn't matter how small this may be. It can be as simple as reading a chapter of a good book, writing a letter, making that phone call you've been looking forward to, watching a television program you've been excited about, or meeting somebody special for lunch. Try to schedule something to look forward to every day. This way, even if part of your day seems boring, whether you're doing menial chores or just resting to build up your strength, you will at least have something enjoyable to look forward to. You won't give the weeds of boredom a chance to take root!

Goal-Setting

Set goals for yourself, both short-term and long-term. Boredom can arise from plodding along with no purpose in life. If you have something specific and tangible to shoot for, you can help fight boredom. This doesn't mean you'll never be bored. You may still have to give yourself an occasional kick in the derriere to keep moving toward these goals. But isn't it better to have something to shoot for than to have nothing at all?

ARE YOU ENVIOUS?

You've heard the cliché, "The grass is always greener..." If you have OA, you are probably envious of others who do not. This is understandable. You may even be envious of other people's joints!

Envy can be a destructive emotion, because it's a type of self-torture. It can be very painful. You constantly put yourself down and compare yourself with the better qualities of somebody else. You feel inferior. This can lead to other feelings as well, such as anger and depression.

Why is envy a problem? Because it shows that you are not satisfied with being yourself. You want to be like somebody else. You want to have what somebody else has. Does this mean that the other person has a happy life? Is that person happier than you in every way? You may have osteoarthritis, but this doesn't mean that everything else about the other person's life is superior. Stop and think for a moment. I'm sure you can come up with some areas in which your life is better!

Is Envy a Positive Emotion?

In general, emotions usually serve a purpose. Emotions such as anger and anxiety mobilize you to prepare to handle their sources. On the other hand, envy is a destructive emotion. It does not have the positive qualities that other emotions have. But maybe you can find something positive in envy. If you recognize that you're envious, analyze the reason why. Try to change your attitude by concentrating on yourself and your own attributes. Don't let envy get you down.

How Does Envy Occur?

Basically, there are four conditions necessary for you to become envious. First, you must feel deprived. You will feel like you can't have something that you want or need. This doesn't mean just money, pleasure, working joints, or even health. Envy is an intense feeling that involves more than this. It'll seem like your feeling of need lies deep inside. Second, somebody else must have whatever it is that you feel you're missing. Third, you must feel powerless to do anything about it. You'll feel totally unable to change the circumstances that made you envious in the first place. This helplessness will cause you to feel more and more bitter—and this will make you even more envious! Fourth, there must be a change in the relationship between you and whatever it is that you envy, be it person, object, or situation. You will no longer simply compare yourself with the other, but will feel fiercely competitive. You may begin to feel that the only reason you don't have what you would like is because somebody else does.

If you feel envious, is it necessarily the same kind of envy that everyone feels? No. There are actually two types of envy. One is an envy of tangible items (cars, boats, homes, friends, and so on). The other is an envy of abstract things, such as pleasure or health. If you have OA, you may still have many tangible things. You may still have a family, a car, and a place to live. You may still have a job. But you tend to be more emotional when you are denied good health than when you are denied a material item. If you have OA, it is natural to be envious of people who are in good health.

What Can You Do?

Concentrate on yourself. Increase the positive benefits and pleasures you can get out of life. Why worry about comparing yourself with somebody else? What's that going to do? Sure, your body may not be functioning the way it used to. But that doesn't mean that you can't enjoy life as much as anybody else can. Set up reasonable goals for yourself, considering other things you have and how you feel. Then you can say that you're living your life as enjoyably as anybody else. This will become easier when you do not compare yourself with somebody else. Remember, you are you. Concentrate on making the best of your own life.

ARE YOU LONELY?

There is a difference between being alone and being lonely. Being alone simply means that there is no one else with you. This can be either good or bad. But being lonely is usually a downer. If you feel lonely, it doesn't really matter whether there's anyone with you. Loneliness is a sad, empty feeling, but one that is usually created by you.

Why might you feel lonely? You may feel left out if you can't spend time with others the way you used to, either because you're not feeling well or because you can't do what others want to do. Maybe you feel lonely because other people don't want to be with you. You may decide to change some of your relationships because you don't want to chance being rejected. Does this mean that you'll be happy about these changes? No.

It's hard to be lonely. Not just because you feel bad, though. It actually takes effort to make yourself lonely—it doesn't just happen. And you have to work hard to keep yourself feeling lonely. There are many opportunities to be with people. As a result, loneliness usually occurs out of choice rather than by accident. In order to be really lonely, you'd have to purposely exclude everyone around you from your life. You'd have to always be on your guard, protecting yourself from the horrible possibility of making a new friend!

Why Be Lonely?

Why might you want to be lonely? There are four reasons. First, if you're lonely, you probably enjoy being lonely. This may contradict your complaints to everyone else. You're lonely because you like it enough not to do anything about it. Second, if you're lonely, it's because you're hard to please. You may feel that you don't want to even bother trying to create new relationships since no one meets all of your requirements. Third, you may be lonely because you feel you must be lonely. You've resigned yourself to it. You tell yourself that this is part of the price you have to pay for having OA! Fourth, and probably most important, you may be lonely because you're afraid. You're afraid to develop new relationships. You're afraid to make yourself vulnerable because you fear rejection. You may recall previous experiences that did not work out the way you wanted. You don't want to relive the hurt and pain.

Break Your Lonely Ways

Reading about this isn't easy, especially if you are a lonely person. Why? It's not easy to believe that you may be doing this yourself! But there is still a light at the end of the tunnel! Recognize where your feelings of loneliness come from. Admit to yourself that loneliness may not be such a great feeling and that you should try to change the way you feel. There are things that you can do.

Don't Be a Pusher

The first step is to stop pushing people away. Your body is sending out signals that tell people that you don't want them around. Your negative body language can reduce your number of acquaintances, adding to your feelings of loneliness. You must stop relaying these messages. You have to learn to give off positive vibrations—the kind that welcome people instead of chasing them away.

Contact!

Once you start giving off new, more positive vibes, you'll want to make more friends. How can you meet people? You can start by getting involved in some kind of organization. This type of activity usually attracts people who are interested in being with others who share a common goal. Because you have OA, you may want to become involved in your local chapter of the Arthritis Foundation. There you'll meet other people with similar concerns (helping you to better cope with your illness). In addition, you may be able to find ways of helping others who have OA. This is a great way to develop friendships.

Try getting involved in a new learning activity or hobby. Take adult education courses, for example. This will help alleviate loneliness as well as boredom. Invite people to your home, but pace yourself so that you don't become exhausted. Most importantly, be receptive to the people that you meet. Try to see the good in everyone. Don't reject someone simply because there are some things about them that you don't like.

If you work at conquering loneliness, you'll feel much better about yourself and about your life. Your life will become more enjoyable, despite your OA. Give yourself and others a chance, and your feelings of loneliness will disappear, regardless of the limitations your condition has placed on you.

ARE YOU UPSET?

Are there times when you are unhappy, but you aren't really depressed? Or when you are uncomfortable but not anxious? You may not know exactly what's bothering you, or what to do about it. Or you may know exactly what's wrong, but you just don't like it. You can do things, but you wish that you could feel better. You may feel mixed up, confused, disturbed, agitated, or shaken. This is typical of feeling upset. Can you get upset because of osteoarthritis? Be serious, now!

When things happen to upset you, you may try to push them out of your mind so that you can adjust as slowly and as comfortably as possible. But eventually, you'll want to come to grips with it.

When you become upset, you're roused to action. Like other emotions, being upset can propel you to do something. So what should you do when you're all motivated? Try to figure out why you're upset, so that you can do something about it. There's probably something in your life that is out of sorts. Things are not moving along smoothly. Something has "upset the apple cart."

Alice was upset. A 55-year-old mother of three, she had just completed her latest shopping trip and was about to relax in front of her favorite soap opera. She had a gnawing feeling that things just weren't right, and this upset her. She knew that she was upset when she found that she couldn't enjoy her program. My goodness, she had been hooked on this show for almost twenty years! But she decided to turn off the TV and figure out what was upsetting her. After at least four commercials' worth of thought, she realized that it was her soap opera that was bothering her! She felt that the characters on the program, despite all of their script problems, were better off than she was. None of them seemed to be experiencing the pain of OA—only she was! None of them needed medication—only she did! None of them needed daily exercises to keep their joints limber. But she did! As she thought about it, however, she realized that perhaps she was making something out of nothing. Actors and actresses have their own problems. So what if she also had something she must learn to live with? Medication and exercise were keeping her condition in check. She might not like it, but she needed it. She quickly noticed that she was feeling much better. In fact, she was able to turn on the television and breathlessly catch the last few minutes of her show!

Once you discover why you are upset, you can act to resolve it. If you can identify what is upsetting you, you can then plan a strategy to eliminate your distress. If you can't figure out what's upsetting you, recognize that you can't and move on.

PART III.
Changes in General Lifestyle

12

Coping With Changes in General Lifestyle—An Introduction

So you have to make changes in some aspects of your lifestyle because of osteoarthritis? Yes, that is all part of the "package." Every time you experience pain when you move, you'll be reminded that things have changed. However, changes may occur in anyone's life for a number of reasons. If you started a new job, you might have to wake up at a different time, travel to work in a new direction by a new form of transportation, or "survive" on a different salary. If your new job required you to move, you would have to meet a whole new group of people. If you bought a new car, you'd have to get used to its gadgets, as well as its quirks.

In your case, OA is a new addition to your life! Although it may be hard for you to try to lead a normal life when you know your condition may never totally be cured, you're not (or shouldn't be) aiming for perfection. You just want to feel better, enjoy life, and do what you can. That's reasonable and achievable.

Why are lifestyle changes such an important part of the treatment program for OA? One of the most important goals of OA management is to relieve or reduce pain. Your lifestyle needs to be altered in order to adapt, reduce, or eliminate those activities that may cause you pain. Changes in lifestyle can also help to prevent more damage to your joints, reducing the chances of developing deformities.

Because osteoarthritis can affect work, family life, sexuality, social activities with friends, finances, and other aspects of daily living, it's important for you to learn how to cope with changes in lifestyle. In some cases, these changes may be minimal. But you might as well understand what you can do to cope with any changes that do occur.

Your lifestyle is of your own choosing. You'll automatically take many different factors into consideration when determining what your lifestyle is and what you want it to be. You can decide how full you want your days to be. You may also decide to put things off until you "feel better." But in the case of osteoarthritis, why wait? Why not try to see what you can do right now to improve the quality of your life, while you're learning to live with OA?

MAKING SOME CHANGES

A good way to change your lifestyle is to look for ways to make things easier for yourself. This may allow you to continue doing much of what you used to do, without putting as much pressure on your body. For people who have problems with joints, everyday activities can put stress and pressure on them. Can these activities be eliminated? Of course not. So the best approach to improving your lifestyle is to find easier ways of doing them.

For example, try to spread out your most taxing activities. Why is it necessary to do all the house cleaning in one day? Spread it out. Pace yourself. Make sure you include rest periods during the course of the day to give your joints a chance to relax. (More about this later.)

As you make changes (at your own pace), you'll feel even better because you'll probably experience less discomfort. You'll make changes in lifestyle that can help you to reduce or avoid your discomfort, save your energy, and protect your joints.

Climate Concerns

Should you move to a different climate? Are certain climates better for osteoarthritis? For years, people have believed that moving to a warm, dry climate could be helpful for OA. It is true that people who retire to such climates, or spend months at a health spa there, may feel better. However, neither the spa nor the climate will necessarily have a significant effect on the course of the disease, although either may be helpful in relieving symptoms. There is no evidence that any specific kind of climate improves or cures osteoarthritis.

Sure, some people may like the idea of moving. It may give them a psychological lift. In some cases, people may feel better after moving to other climates. But then again, this is true for people who don't have OA, as well!

In order to decide if such a move should occur, you must consider the emotional and financial effects of such a change. You'll have to change jobs, find a new place to live, and possibly even adopt a new lifestyle. You'll be leaving old family and friends behind (of course, this may be a blessing in disguise if you're leaving behind people who deserve to be left behind!).

You have to weigh the advantages of moving (such as the possibility of feeling more comfortable) and the disadvantages (such as disrupting your family). If you really are contemplating a geographical change, it's probably a good idea to take an extended vacation in that location before actually committing yourself to such a move. If a move is going to help you to feel better, you'll probably realize this during your extended vacation. But remember: on a vacation, you don't have to cook, clean, or participate in many of the other joyful chores of life. You may feel better only because of less stress and less wear and tear. However, once you move, you'll have a home to fix up and a family to care for, among other responsibilities, so stress may recur.

GETTING USED TO THE CHANGES

What are some of the factors that will determine how well you'll adapt to changes in your lifestyle? There are many. For example, what were you doing before you started experiencing OA discomfort? How satisfied were you with your major vocational (job) and avocational (leisure or recreation) activities? How much education did you have? How supportive were the people close to you—both family and friends? How has your condition affected you, both physically and emotionally? These and other questions play a role in determining how you'll adjust to OA, its treatment, and the changes it necessitates. But that doesn't mean your hands will be tied. You can improve the way you deal with virtually every aspect of osteoarthritis.

Yes, there will be some changes in your lifestyle. But why assume that all of them have to be negative? Isn't it possible that some of them might be for the better? Maybe you were such a hard worker that you never spent enough time with your family. If you have to cut back on your work schedule because of OA, perhaps you'll enjoy the increased time you'll have to spend with your family. Learning to take better care of yourself will pay off in the long run. So don't convince yourself that your life is ruined just because your joints are giving you a hard time! Always look at the positive in any situation.

We'll be discussing how to deal with as many of the negatives as possible.

Your head may be spinning, fearing changes that may have to take place in your activity schedule, job, or social relationships. You may also be apprehensive about dealing with physical discomfort, body changes, and medication, to name only a few areas of concern. In fact,you may even be worried that you won't be able to perform your normal chores and responsibilities. This fear is not unusual. Most people with OA do feel this way. But feelings will improve. Realizing that you can do more will also help to improve your spirits.

How About Denial?

What happens if you decide not to accept necessary changes in lifestyle? This may indicate that you're trying to deny your problem. Denial is a very common coping strategy. But believe it or not, denial can be a positive technique. How? It can help by keeping you from dwelling on problems that aren't helped by dwelling! But denial has its negative side, too. What if denial keeps you from doing what you need to do? For example, what if you don't get enough rest, or you're too active, or, or, or. . . ? This is *destructive denial*, and it can hurt you. Hopefully, the fact that you're reading this book in the first place shows that you're not really denying inappropriately. But continue to stay on top of this.

TIPS FOR CHANGE

Here are some general tips for living with OA that make sense if you need to modify your lifestyle:

- Try to plan activities in advance. Make sure that strenuous activity is limited. Avoid excessive physical and emotional fatigue and strain.
- Any time your chores cause you discomfort, try to figure out ways to make things easier for yourself. Reorganize rooms, work areas, and other parts of your home (and life) to maximize efficiency and convenience.
- Try to arrange your tasks so that they flow naturally and easily from one to the other. For example, try to avoid trips back and forth to different rooms of the house.
- Try to avoid carrying. When shopping, make use of shopping

carts or use bags to carry items, rather than holding them in your hands.

- Try to avoid excessive bending, straining, or reaching. Sit if you can, rather than standing.
- Take frequent breaks while driving. It's not good to sit or hold your head in one position for too long. And make sure you have "healthy" shock absorbers in your car. They can reduce the bounce and motion, and help your own shock absorbers feel better!
- Try to avoid sitting on too soft a seat. If you start feeling uncomfortable, get up and walk around.
- Try to read or watch TV while sitting in a chair. You can strain your neck doing these activities in bed.
- Use support devices when appropriate in order to save unnecessary work or activity.
- Always alternate rest periods with prolonged periods of activity. For example, you might want to plan on ten minutes of rest for each hour of activity.
- Learn your "pain threshold." If you know when you have reached the limit of how much pain you want to endure, you can slow down or stop, give your joints a rest, and not chance damaging them.

Coping with changes in lifestyle forms a very important part of the process we call rehabilitation. What is your goal? To help yourself to live as satisfying a life as possible despite your condition.

The rest of this book will address many of your concerns about lifestyle changes. The remaining chapters of Part III will be concerned primarily with changes in the way your body feels, the way OA affects you, and the things you do. So read on, and let's get your act together!

13

Physical Changes

Unfortunately, there may be some physical changes in your body because of OA. Although effective management may stop or slow down the progression of OA, it may not reverse damage that has already occurred. So physical changes can take place and affect how well you adjust psychologically to your condition.

What can you do? Well, you won't be able to do something about all the physical changes, but many of them can be helped. So first concentrate on those things you *can* do something about. Then work on learning how to accept and live with the ones you can't change. That may seem like a tall order, but what choice do you have? After all, you're still the same person inside, aren't you (and I'm not talking about your joints!)?

Let's discuss two of the more common physical changes that may occur with OA—fatigue and joint problems—and how to better cope with them. (Pain has a chapter all to itself!) Is there anything you can do about these changes? Several suggestions will be offered. If you can't use them, at least you'll be learning more about the changes, and you'll become aware that you're not alone in experiencing them.

FATIGUE

Do you become tired more easily? Does your bed seem to be your favorite place in the whole world? If so, you're not alone. Fatigue (yawn!) is a very common problem for individuals with OA, although it is caused more by the pain of the disease than by the disease itself. Your entire body reflects the pain you're feeling. You're more tense, you hold yourself differently, and you move differently. Whew! Exhausting! You may find that simply getting up, washing, and getting dressed makes you tired. You may be pooped for the rest of the day.

Fatigue can be caused by doing *too* much! Or it can occur even if you haven't been too active. In this case, the fatigue can be due to other factors such as emotions, anemia, or medication. And, of course, haven't you often said, "I'm sick and *tired* of this pain!"?

Consider the possibility that your fatigue may be emotional rather than physical. In other words, you're tired because of the way you feel emotionally—not so much because of physical exhaustion. If this is the case, try to determine what emotional reactions are contributing to the fatigue. For example, fatigue could be due to depression, boredom, worry, or just unhappiness. After you discover what is causing your fatigue, you can work on improving these feelings.

Most people think of fatigue as negative. This is not always the case. It can be positive. How? Fatigue is your body's way of telling you that you need rest. If you didn't feel tired, you would push yourself too much! Then you'd probably feel even more pain. So if you feel fatigue, you should listen to your body.

What Can You Do?

What's the best way to cope with fatigue? Rest. (Clever!) A good night's sleep or short naps during the day are great for coping with fatigue.

Although rest may not make your fatigue disappear, it can certainly help. If fatigue is a message that your body is unable to do as much as you want it to do, rest is certainly an important way to gain more control. One problem, however, is that *too much rest* can lead to more fatigue! This can start a vicious cycle.

Fatigue can also be reduced by efficient planning and pacing. Figure out what you have to do. Schedule activities so that you're not doing too many strenuous things in a row. Make sure you intersperse rest periods with any strenuous activities you need to do. And be flexible. You can never be sure when you're going to have energy, or when you're going to feel too tired to do anything.

Know your priorities. Focus on the top priorities while you still have the energy. That way, if fatigue sets in, you will need to delay only the less significant activities.

Other techniques that you will learn while becoming an "efficiency expert," such as reorganizing your house to make things more convenient, will also help you to do more and feel less fatigued. Don't feel as if you have to make all these changes by yourself.

Professionals can give you advice that may help to improve how well you function day to day.

JOINT PROBLEMS

Joint problems are the main physical complaint in osteoarthritis. Other than pain, stiffness (especially in the morning) is a very common characteristic of OA. After awakening in the morning and after sitting or standing still for a short period of time, your body may stiffen up. Fortunately, this is usually of short duration. After a brief period of loosening up, movement may become easier and less painful.

What Can You Do?

The primary treatment for joint problems involves medication and physical therapy (both discussed in Chapters 14 and 15). But there are other things that can be done, too.

Supportive devices such as canes, crutches, walkers, splints, or braces can help those joints in the hands, ankles, feet, hips, or knees. They preserve and protect them (sounds like the U.S. Constitution!) and allow for as much functional mobility as possible. These devices may also help by spreading out the weight that would be placed on any weight-bearing joints.

What can be done about joint stiffness? Remember that one of the best ways to treat morning stiffness is to treat your OA in general. It's possible that you haven't been taking proper care of yourself, and stiffness may serve as a reminder. Try to loosen up slowly, gradually, and gently, but recognize that it may still take a little time for your joints to become more mobile. Make sure you're taking medication at the proper times.

A warm (not hot) bath or shower may be helpful. Gentle exercises may help to loosen you up. Anticipate that you will experience a certain amount of stiffness each day. Work it out of your joints as comfortably as you can.

Principles of Joint Protection

You'll want to do everything you can to protect your joints from further damage or stress. Some medication may even work better if you protect an affected joint from excessive motion or from bearing too much weight. So it can be very helpful to become aware of some of the basic principles of joint protection.

- Try to use the strongest or largest joint possible when you have to do something. For example, your wrist is a larger joint than your fingers. Therefore, when possible, use your wrist instead of using your fingers. In the same vein, try using your shoulder instead of your elbow, and so on.
- Try to avoid placing too much pressure against small joints of the hand (such as the backs or pads of your fingers). This can put too much stress on the weakened joints to the knuckles. Use your palms instead of your fingers whenever possible.
- Try not to allow joints to remain in one particular position for too long. In other words, if you have to hold something—whether it's a cup, glass, book, or cards—try not to hold it in the same position for too long. Change positions as often as you can (within reason).
- Try to extend your joints as much as possible in all activities. People with joint problems tend to keep them slightly contracted (flexed). Why? A slight contraction of the joints is usually more comfortable if you're in pain, or even if a joint is normal. This is because flexing makes use of stronger muscles than extension. Extending your joints (opening them fully) can keep joints mobile even though it may be slightly less comfortable when you do so. Interestingly enough, extended joints may require less strain.
- Avoid lifting whenever you possibly can, for it is a very stressful activity.

A PHYSICAL FINALE

So there are changes as a result of OA. This chapter has included only the two most common ones. You may not be thrilled with them. But once again, what's the alternative? You do want to learn how to cope with OA and the changes that result from it. That's why you're reading this book, right?

14

Pain

Ouch! (Just getting you ready for this chapter!) Is osteoarthritis painful? Are you kidding?! Most individuals with OA believe that the pain is the hardest thing to deal with. But the good news is that treatment for OA is designed to improve the quality of your life and decrease your discomfort.

What is pain? Pain is a type of sensation picked up by nerve endings and transmitted to the brain. This message is very important. Why? Pain is a signal from your body telling you that you're having trouble in a particular part. In OA, it can tell you that a joint is injured or that you're using a damaged joint too much. It also signals you to "slow down" to prevent additional damage. As a result, pain can be an important diagnostic tool. Only *you* know the intensity of your pain. Pain suggests that you rest the injured areas of your body so that your tissues can be repaired. It can help you to determine the nature or severity of an illness or injury. Only after these messages travel from the site of irritation to the brain do we feel pain.

What can you do about your discomfort? How can you cope with it? The best way to cope with pain is to get rid of it! To do this, it's first necessary to identify the cause of the pain.

CAUSES OF YOUR PAIN

Although it's still not completely understood what causes the pain of OA, it's generally believed that the pain results when the nerves in the joint become irritated. The pain of OA may be caused by changes in a joint's bone structure, or by pressure on the nerves by osteophytes. Stiffness and tenderness also contribute to the pain. Inflammation and swelling can be painful as well because of the pressure created.

Besides the pressure, tension and spasm in muscles or fatigue can also be contributors.

Earlier in the development of OA, pain may be triggered only by movement. Eventually, however, pain may increase to the point where it might occur during rest periods as well.

GETTING STARTED

Once you're aware of what's causing your pain, treatment can attempt to eliminate the cause. But what if you can't do anything about the underlying source of the pain? At least you can try to get some relief from it.

How do you start? First, be aware of your pain. While this may sound strange, you'll learn to recognize whether your pain is something you can (and should) handle yourself, or if it's serious enough to be discussed with your doctor. Remember: If in doubt, check it out. Inform your doctor about the pain. Because pain is different for each person, you'll want to recognize when you're in pain that needs attention, and when you can handle it. You'll also want to be able to distinguish between pain and stiffness, and be familiar with the pattern of your pain. All of these things will help you and your doctor work out the best ways of dealing with it.

WHEN DOES PAIN OCCUR?

Many factors may contribute to your pain. You'll want to try to control any or all of these factors in order to manage it. Remember that pain can be affected by both psychological and environmental factors. Although pain may initially be physical, emotions can quickly worsen or exacerbate the pain. So pain may result from stress, fatigue, or depression.

Stress causes you to tense your muscles. It may make it more difficult for you to relax, and can increase the degree of pain that you're experiencing. If you're fatigued, you may feel more pain because your tissues and joints aren't getting the rest they need to repair themselves. Depression may cause you to feel more pain too, because your OA is frequently on your mind.

When you're in pain, this may increase the degree to which you experience stress, fatigue, or depression. This can lead to more pain, creating a vicious cycle.

TREATMENT FOR PAIN

There are four traditional categories of therapy for pain control: chemical (using medication), surgical, physical (physical therapy), and psychological. In general, all four therapies work by interrupting the transmission of pain messages before the brain receives and interprets them.

Medical treatment for pain generally involves medication. This can effectively control a lot of problems. For example, aspirin has been proven effective in controlling minor pain. But sometimes discomfort will continue, despite the use of medication. (The next chapter will go into much more detail on medication.) In extreme cases, surgery may be helpful in treating the cause of the pain. But not all conditions lend themselves to surgical treatment. So it may be necessary for you to learn other techniques for dealing with pain.

Other than medicine and surgery, what are other ways of trying to obtain pain relief? Physical therapy techniques (such as using TENS units, heat, cold, hydrotherapy, and a proper balance of rest and exercise) can be used, as well as psychological techniques such as imagery, biofeedback, yoga, hypnosis, and relaxation. (More about these later.) Last but not least, it's very important to maintain a positive attitude.

You can learn how to employ techniques for controlling pain from physicians, physical therapists, occupational therapists, and mental health professionals (such as psychologists who may specialize in certain pain control techniques). Or you may want to read some of the many books on pain which can be found in bookstores and libraries. A good book to read is *Free Yourself From Pain* by David Breslin. Another one is *Life Without Pain* by Richard Linchitz.

Many techniques for pain control can be applied at home, although in some cases they may achieve greater success in clinics or centers.

Despite the effectiveness of the pain control techniques mentioned in this chapter, it's important to consult your physician to make sure that any or all the techniques are appropriate for you. Make sure that any techniques that you're thinking of using will not be dangerous for you, considering your condition.

Now let's go on to discuss some of these techniques.

TENS Units

TENS stands for Transcutaneous Electrical Nerve Stimulation. These devices have been gaining in popularity to help control pain. The TENS unit is a little box about the size of a cigarette pack. It contains a generator that has wire leads with electrodes at the ends of them. The unit may have anywhere from two to forty electrode wire leads. A little gel is attached to the electrodes. They're then placed on your skin, on or near the area to be treated. When you turn on the unit, a low level of electricity flows into the area from the TENS unit. This stimulates the nerve fibers and blocks the transmission of pain messages to the brain. Shocking, right? Don't worry. You probably won't even feel anything, or you may just experience a mild tingling sensation.

One of the problems with TENS units is that their effectiveness seems to decrease as time goes by. The effectiveness of the TENS units also seems to be related to your diligence, the knowledge of your therapist, and the appropriate placing of electrodes.

If you want to get a TENS unit, you usually need a prescription from your physician. You can then be taught by a nurse or physical therapist how to place the electrodes to provide you with maximum pain relief. But it's probably a good idea to rent a machine before buying one to see if it works for you.

Heat and Cold

Both heat and cold treatments can be beneficial in the temporary relief of painful OA symptoms. However, neither has an effect on the disease itself. If you're going to use either heat or cold, be careful! You can hurt yourself if you misuse it.

Some people seem to benefit more from heat; others seem to benefit more from cold. This may vary within you as well, depending upon the stage of your disease. There may be times when they work best in combination. At other times, different joints may benefit from different approaches.

Heat

Heat can be a very beneficial way of relaxing and soothing your muscles to relieve soreness and pain. This is called thermotherapy. It's considered to be the oldest form of pain reliever or analgesic.

Heat increases the temperature in a selected area of your body. There are two good reasons for this. One: It increases blood circulation to the area. Two: It increases the metabolic rate.

If you're using heat, you should feel comfortably warmed and relaxed. By relaxing tight muscles, you can increase the mobility of your joint. (This is one reason why using heat before exercise can be helpful.) Usually, positive effects from heat can be felt in about twenty minutes, give or take a few minutes. However, trial and error is necessary to find out what's best for you.

Is Heat Always Helpful?

Heat may not always be appropriate. If an affected joint is treated with heat, it may aggravate symptoms in this joint. For example, there may be increased swelling or damage. Heat may be harder to tolerate if you're very young or very old.

If you are going to use heat, be careful about the intensity and duration of its use. Too much heat for too long a period of time is not advisable. Don't assume that if a little bit of heat is good, a lot of heat can be better. This is a good way to get burned!

Ways to Apply Heat

The methods of applying heat may be divided into two categories: moist heat and dry heat. Examples of moist heat include using hot towels (or hydrocollators), hydrotherapy, or water baths. Hydrotherapy can be used for both hot and cold applications. (More about this later.) Dry heat can be applied using heating pads, lamps, or heaters. (Obviously, if you use any electrical appliances, use them carefully!)

Is there a difference between the effectiveness of moist heat and dry heat? Not very much. Both can be effective as long as the frequency, duration of treatment, and intensity are controlled.

Some ways of applying heat may be more effective for large areas of your body; others may be more effective for small areas. Let's discuss some specific heat treatment techniques.

Hydrocollators. One way to apply moist heat is by using warm, damp towels or hydrocollators. Hydrocollators may be very helpful in relieving pain and reducing inflammation. What is a hydrocollator? The hydrocollator pack is usually made up of a canvas sack that contains a gel. That's why it may also be called a "gel pack." It is heated in hot water, wrapped in terry cloth, and applied to the painful area for about twenty minutes. The silica gel contained in the hydrocollator pack can retain heat for a long period of time. Or you can make your own hot compresses of towels. This involves soaking a towel in hot water, then wringing it out and applying it to the painful area.

If you use hydrocollator packs or hot compresses, be careful to avoid burns! In general, a good way to avoid burns and retain heat for longer periods of time is to use plastic sheets or dry towels wrapped around the hot compress.

Warm Baths. A warm bath in the morning is a great idea. Not only can it be very helpful in reducing the stiffness and pain you'll feel upon awakening, but you'll get clean in the bargain! Hot showers can also reduce stiffness. Many muscles can be relaxed at the same time. Usually baths or showers should last no longer than twenty minutes. Why? They may make you tired, even in that short period of time.

Paraffin Wax Treatments. Paraffin wax treatments, using melted wax, is a good way to apply heat to the hands. (Make sure you initially use these treatments under the supervision of your doctor or physical therapist.) Usually, the painful area is dipped in melted wax ten to twelve times. This forms a very thin, glove-like layer that covers the area, coats it, and keeps it warm for a fairly long period of time. Once the wax is in place, the joints must remain still or else the wax will crack. After fifteen to forty-five minutes, the wax is peeled off. Because of the close adhesion of the wax to the body, it's not a good idea to use paraffin treatments on body parts that contain open wounds. It's also important to be very careful while heating the wax, to avoid fire hazards.

Heating Pads. Electric heating pads can be helpful but should not be used for long periods of time. They should be placed on top of the painful area. It's not a good idea to lay on a heating pad or sleep with one on. Heating pads are usually safest at low settings.

An electric blanket may also be helpful. Not only does it provide warmth, which can be soothing to your joints, but it also means that you'll require fewer blankets in cold weather. So what, you say? Well, if you need fewer blankets, you won't have to bear the weight of a large number of blankets on your already weakened joints! Get it?

Heat Lamps. Heat lamps (diathermy) can be useful for small parts of the body. Infrared bulbs are the best bulbs to use, not ultraviolet bulbs like those found in sunlamps. You want to help your pain, not tan your skin!

Cold

Although there are many benefits to using heat treatments, some people and situations respond better to cold treatment. Cold treatments, also known as cryotherapy, can help the painful joints of OA. How? Cold has a numbing effect on nerve endings in the affected areas. It also decreases the activity of the body cells.

One common method of cold treatment involves soaking a cloth or towel in ice water, wringing it out, and applying it to the painful area. As with hot compresses, you can protect yourself and prolong the effectiveness of the treatment by using plastic sheets or dry towels. Another type of cold compress can be made by wrapping a towel around a plastic bag that has been filled with ice cubes. Cold treatments can also involve commercially available chemical cold packs, but this can get expensive if you're purchasing packs that are not reusable.

Some people don't like cold treatments, saying that they're only good for polar bears. Others, however, find that greater pain relief can be obtained by using cold rather than heat treatments.

Contrast Baths

Contrast baths may be helpful in relieving pain and swelling for some individuals. If you use them, you will be contrasting hot and cold water treatments. The most common procedure used for contrast baths is to soak the extremities alternately for three minutes in hot water (at approximately 110°F) and one minute in cold water (at approximately 65°F).

Hydrotherapy

Hydrotherapy, or water baths, may be a very helpful way to get your joints more mobile, as well as to promote relaxation, improve deep breathing, increase circulation, reduce extremity swelling, and improve coordination. Hydrotherapy can also be helpful as a heat technique.

But hydrotherapy can cause fatigue, so it should not be done for a long period of time. And there should be somebody there with you, if possible.

Pool Exercise Programs

Pool exercise programs, also called "aquatics" by the Arthritis Foundation, can be very beneficial for your OA. (They can also be helpful if you don't have the disease!) You can exercise many parts of your body in the water. Exercising in pools is safe and much less strenuous than the same exercise outside of water. It can also be enjoyable! You're more likely to build up the strength of your muscles and range of motion in your joints when you're in the water. It's possible to do much more in water than out of the water. Movements are easier in the water because weight is relieved by its buoyancy. You'll be able to more easily move joints that are weakened and painful. The warmth tends to reduce the pain and spasms of muscles.

You may find that you feel better about yourself because you're able to move more normally in the water. As a result, you can exercise for a longer period of time.

There are many centers that have specific aquatics exercise programs for individuals with arthritis. Check with your local chapter of the Arthritis Foundation for further details.

Alleviating the Pain Psychologically

Is pain purely physiological? Rarely. It's usually a combination of physiological and psychological factors. What does this mean? Although your joints may be hurting, it's your *mind* that determines just how much it hurts.

Angela was moving exceptionally slowly, primarily because she had a lot of pain in her knees. The pain overwhelmed her every time she tried to move faster. Even when she was doing something she enjoyed, her movements were restricted. Suddenly, she heard her 6-year-old son cry out for help. Without thinking about her joint pain, she went flying across the room to help him. How could her pain have been purely physiological? Yes, Angela had been in pain, but her mind had probably magnified it. When she had realized that her son was in trouble, her pain had temporarily taken on secondary importance.

What does all this mean? If medication or other medical intervention doesn't help alleviate your pain, you can still relieve some (if not all) of it by working on your mind's awareness of it. Read on to find out how you can do this.

Relaxation Techniques

Relaxation can be helpful in controlling pain. Relaxation is the opposite of tension, which can actually increase your pain. Relaxation is also helpful in loosening the muscles that may contribute to your pain. There are a number of different types of relaxation procedures including meditation, autogenic training, hypnosis, and deep breathing procedures.

Let's discuss other psychological techniques to help control pain, such as imagery, biofeedback, and changing your way of thinking.

Imagery

There is a relationship between your mind and the way you feel physically. Much research has proven this. Scientists have also found that bodily functions, previously thought to be totally beyond conscious control (autonomic is the scientific term), can be modified using psychological techniques! One such technique is imagery, or the process of conjuring up pictures or scenes in your mind. In practice, imagery has been beneficial in helping to deal with a host of physiological and psychological problems, including headaches, hypertension, depression, and pain. In many cases, imagery procedures have worked well in combination with prescribed medication for treating illness.

Here's how imagery works. Sit in a comfortable chair or in bed and get into a relaxed position. Lights should be dimmed, and outside sounds or noises minimized, with no interruptions. Breathe smoothly and rhythmically, allowing your body to release tension and relax. Then imagine a scene of your own choosing, trying to make the image as vivid and real as possible. This scene can be used therapeutically to help you feel better.

Anita was suffering from a sharp pain in her knees. She was instructed to relax and then develop an image of what this joint looked like. She imagined it as a very sharp knife jabbed into her knees. Others may feel like their knees are being hit by a hammer or have dozens of pins stuck into them. Whatever imagery you develop, it should be as vivid and detailed as possible. Anita was then instructed to reverse what was happening in the image: She imagined the knife slowly being removed from the knees, and a soothing cream being applied. Finally, the knife was completely out. She was then able to relax and her discomfort was eliminated.

There are other images you could use to reduce joint pain. For example, you could imagine oil or a soothing lotion being gently massaged into the affected joint, or you could picture yourself taking a warm bath. These images can be used anywhere. (Have you ever taken a bath on a bus?!) With regular use, they can help you feel better. Imagery is really enhanced by your creativity. A good book on the subject is *In the Mind's Eye* by Arnold Lazarus. See if your public library or local bookstore has it.

Imagery is also a key component in hypnosis. You might choose to use hypnosis, since it can be helpful in pain control.

Biofeedback

Biofeedback combines the procedures of relaxation and imagery with the use of measuring instruments—usually electronic ones. These machines let you know what's going on physiologically (giving you feedback) in your body (bio). The devices, which are connected to different parts of your body, provide moment-by-moment information about any changes that are taking place.

Biofeedback can help you learn to control certain automatic body functions by obtaining feedback from certain measurement techniques. You can learn how to voluntarily control internal functions of your body that you may have previously thought were involuntary or uncontrollable. Blood flow and activities of the brain are among the body's automatic functions.

One of the main advantages of biofeedback is that there are usually signals that you can hear or see. Electrodes are either taped to your skin or attached in some other way. They pick up responses that are transmitted to the biofeedback unit as electrical impulses. These impulses are then translated into sounds or lights that you can observe. In this way, you may receive continuous information about body functions such as blood pressure, heart rate, muscle tension, or skin temperature. Using this information, you can develop different types of imagery so that you can learn how to control your internal responses.

Glenda was experiencing a lot of joint pain in her shoulder, so her physician suggested she try biofeedback. A machine measuring muscle tension was attached to her shoulder (in much the same way that electrodes from an EKG machine are connected. There is no pain, and you won't get jolted!). As she attempted to relax, the machine gave her instant feedback as to whether she was really relaxing, and to what degree. As she became aware of her lowering tension, she learned what mental images were helping her to relax. She could then continue using these images on her own, without the machine, to help her relax and control some of the pain.

What kinds of biofeedback equipment may be used? Most frequently, machines can be used to measure skin temperature, pulse, blood pressure, electrical activity resulting from muscular tension, or electrical activity coming from the brain.

There are some people who wonder whether biofeedback does anything other than help you to relax your muscles. Further research is still necessary.

Not much research has been done specifically on the effects of biofeedback on arthritis patients. However, research has indicated that biofeedback can teach you how to relax and help you to control pain, warm hands, and get your muscles to work effectively. This may be helpful for individuals with OA.

Coping Psychologically

There are other factors that can contribute to the intensity (even the very existence) of your pain, including your emotional state, the attention you pay to your pain, and the way the rest of your body feels. Obviously, as you pinpoint which of these factors does play a role, you can begin improving the way you cope with pain.

Where do you start? You'll want to do everything you can to decrease fear, stress, tension, and other negative emotional factors. All of these may make you more aware of your painful physical state. Anything you can do to relieve anxiety and tension (including psychotherapy, if necessary) should help you to cope better with any pain.

How do you reduce the amount of attention focused on your pain? Of course, the more time you have to think about it, the worse it will seem. So try to divert your attention. Develop other interests that require concentration. You can always come up with pleasant thoughts or activities that will distract you from painful thoughts. One very helpful "activity" might be to get involved with a support group for people living with pain. One such organization is the National Chronic Pain Outreach. They have many chapters throughout the country, and more are always forming. It can be great to know that you're not alone in trying to cope with pain. Who knows? You may even get some great ideas that will help to reduce the pain you have to live with!

AN UNAGONIZING CONCLUSION

Whether your pain comes from OA, from your treatment, or from something else, don't throw in the heating pad! Realize that the pain need not last forever. A lot can be done, both medically and psychologically, to help deal with it.

15

Medication

Believe it or not, some people welcome drugs as a powerful way to control problems in the body. Others are afraid of their power and of eventually becoming dependent on them. Still others resent the presence of any artificial substances in their bodies. Where do your feelings fit in? Regardless of what your attitudes are toward using medication, your physician has probably made it perfectly clear that you don't have much choice in the matter. One of the components of a comprehensive treatment program for OA is taking medication. This can help you to live a more comfortable life. How? Medication for OA is prescribed to reduce pain, to help you feel better, and to keep your joints moving! Regardless of how important your medication is, you must remember to take it properly. Otherwise it can be very dangerous.

WHAT TO TAKE

How is it determined which medication is going to be used? Physicians need to be aware of the severity of your OA, the amount of pain you're experiencing, what other drugs you're taking, how well you take what you're supposed to take, and your age and overall health, among other factors. But even when all these factors are taken into consideration, doctors are still not sure exactly how certain medication will affect you. So in many cases, trial and error is necessary in order to determine the proper dosage. You may need to try different kinds of medication over long periods of time in order to arrive at the combination that can best help your condition. This may be very frustrating, but the results are worthwhile. Make sure you understand exactly why you're taking medication and what it's supposed to do.

HOW AND WHEN TO TAKE

Besides knowing *what* medication you're taking and *why* you're taking it, you should completely understand *when* and *how* to take it. For example, certain medications should be taken after meals. Others may be taken during a meal. Still others have to be taken on an empty stomach. Some medication should be taken with water, some with food, and some in other ways.

So far, you know the "what" (which medication you are taking), "why" you are taking it, and "when" and "how" you are to take it. But you also need to know "how much" to take and "how often" to take it. (It seems like "where" to take your medication is really the only thing that's left up to you!) The "how much" and "how often," of course, will be supplied by your physician, but you'll still want to understand why. Each person has different needs as far as dose and frequency are concerned. What somebody else takes may not necessarily be appropriate for you, even if this person seems to share the same problems. The dosage and frequency of the medication can also be based on the reaction you have to it, how well it's doing what it's supposed to do, and the severity of the problem that is being treated.

Once you begin taking medication in certain dosages, don't attempt to change them on your own. Because of the chemical natures of these drugs and the way they may interact in your body, it's extremely important that you follow your doctor's orders when taking the drugs prescribed for you. Don't mix drugs without knowing if the combination is safe. If you need to take many different pills, make sure that you don't play with your dosage, or play with the times you take them, or move around the number of pills you take at a particular time. Follow your doctor's prescription as carefully as possible.

You probably want to take as little medication as possible. Very few physicians will keep you on high doses of any medication unless they feel it's absolutely essential. If you're taking a substantial dose of any drug, then there must be a reason for it. Don't be afraid to ask your doctor about it. Every good doctor will gladly explain your prescribed medication and why you need it.

SIDE EFFECTS

Taking medication for OA may be necessary. But that doesn't necessarily mean you're thrilled, right? Not too many people are. What might bother you? Well, you're probably concerned about what the medication may be doing to your body, or what the side effects may be. This is probably one of the biggest problems concerning medication. Side effects are the "less than pleasant" consequences. They indicate that a drug is interacting with your body in a way other than the way it was intended. Because medication causes chemical changes within the body, side effects may occur whenever medication is taken. Unfortunately, the more powerful the drug, the more potent the side effects. However, remember that the benefits to your body are usually much more important than any potential side effects. Otherwise, your doctor wouldn't prescribe the medication. Physicians are aware of possible side effects; they won't prescribe any medication that isn't necessary (nor at higher dosages than are necessary). If side effects do have a particularly harsh impact on you, then your physician may have to weigh the advantages against the disadvantages. Be aware, however, that the "side effects" of *not* following prescribed treatments may include pain, stiffness, or joint damage, among other problems.

It is important that you take your medication exactly the way it was prescribed for you. Also, you should report any difficulties that you experience with your medication to your physician. (More about specific side effects later in this chapter.)

GETTING DOWN TO SPECIFICS

Let's talk about some of the medication taken for OA. The goal? You want to learn all about any medicine you have to take as part of your life, so that you can cope with the changes. Fortunately, many people with OA only need one type of medication. But, because medications work differently for different people, there are a lot of different kinds out there!

Some of the medication that has been helpful in treating OA can be divided into four main categories:

- Aspirin
- Non-steroidal anti-inflammatory drugs (NSAIDs)
- Other Analgesics (to relieve pain)
- Corticosteroids

Let's look at these different medications closely.

Aspirin

Aspirin is part of the family of salicylates, and is considered the most important drug in the world. That's a pretty bold statement (but true!). Although it's considered a safe and effective drug, it is a powerhouse. Aspirin often begins (and sometimes is the only) drug therapy for osteoarthritis. One of the reasons that aspirin is so important is that it (along with other NSAIDs that we'll discuss soon) has the unique quality of being both a painkiller and an anti-inflammatory.

Virtually every American family has aspirin in its medicine chest at home. However, if aspirin is going to be used as part of treatment for osteoarthritis, it should not be on a self-prescribed basis. It can be very harmful if not taken carefully. You should use medication for your treatment only if it is prescribed and supervised by your doctor.

How Does It Work?

How does aspirin "know" whether it will simply be an analgesic to control pain or if it will also act as an anti-inflammatory? The answer is in the dosage! At low dosages, aspirin can help to reduce pain. How? It acts on the central nervous system and reduces your ability to feel pain. But if aspirin is going to be effective in reducing inflammation, a higher dosage is needed. Why? Higher levels of aspirin are necessary to block the production of substances called prostaglandins. These are the chemicals that help trigger and prolong the inflammatory process. You will experience inflammation in those joints where prostaglandins have been released. These prostaglandins seem to increase the pain you experience because they sensitize nerve endings. Since aspirin interferes with the production of prostaglandins, it also blocks pain and reduces inflammation.

What Dosage?

The correct dosage of aspirin is the one that you can best tolerate. In other words, you should try to keep the dosage of aspirin just below the level at which unpleasant side effects (such as nausea or ringing in the ears) occur. The number of aspirin tablets that people take varies. There is no "correct formula."

Will you need to take aspirin all the time? It depends on how OA is affecting you. If you're using aspirin as an anti-inflammatory, you'll need to maintain high doses for it to work. On the other hand, if you are taking aspirin just to relieve pain, you'll only need to use it when you're in pain. (That makes sense!) Since your life with OA can be pain-free from time to time, you can also be aspirin-free when that occurs!

Fortunately, aspirin is not an addictive drug. Nor does it seem to lose its effectiveness over time. Although some people find that taking a particular medication often enough leads to a need for more of it to do the same job, it doesn't seem to work that way with aspirin.

Should you take generic aspirin? Most physicians feel that there is nothing wrong with this. As a matter of fact, they may advise you to do so because you will save on costs and still get the same quality. What if you were doing well on a brand name aspirin, but you began to flare up when you switched to a generic aspirin? It could be that the generic aspirin has less strength and effectiveness than your brand name aspirin.

Side Effects

There are possible side effects to taking aspirin. Unfortunately, stomach upset is a common side effect of aspirin. You may also experience nausea or indigestion. Vomiting may occur. Usually, taking aspirin with food, milk, or an antacid may alleviate some of these side effects. Sometimes these side effects can be avoided by using special types of coated aspirin. Liquid aspirin or time-release aspirin may also help to avoid an upset stomach, as may buffered aspirin or aspirin mixed with antacids.

Another side effect from high doses of aspirin is tinnitus, a ringing or buzzing in the ears. Dizziness, slight losses of hearing, or slight changes in vision may also result from high levels of aspirin. Aspirin can also cause a small degree of blood loss from the stomach. While not indicating that an ulcer is present, these surface "erosions" from aspirin can lead to a low red blood cell count (anemia). Black stool may be a sign of blood loss. Sometimes, lightheadedness, increased fatigue, and pallor may indicate that anemia is present. However, when aspirin dosage is lowered or stopped, these side effects practically always go away. But please tell your doctor if any of these symptoms occur.

Any Problems?

There are some people who should not take aspirin. Some asthma sufferers may not be able to tolerate it. Aspirin can cause serious bleeding and, on rare occasions, may even lead to hemorrhaging. People with gastrointestinal problems should always use great caution if told to take aspirin. People who are using other types of medication, such as blood thinners, may also be advised to avoid aspirin.

People who are allergic to aspirin (although this does not occur very often) must avoid it. There is a difference between side effects and allergies. If you are allergic to aspirin, you must eliminate this drug from your treatment program; however, if you are experiencing side effects, you may still be able to use it by adjusting your dosage. Symptoms that indicate an allergic reaction include a rash, a runny nose, and wheezing. On the other hand, symptoms such as ringing in the ears, headache, nausea, abdominal pain, and stomach upset are simply side effects.

Why is it so important that you recognize the possible side effects of aspirin? If you are taking aspirin for a long period of time, it is possible you will develop some of these side effects. If this occurs, talk to your doctor. You may be advised to reduce your dosage slightly, in order to determine exactly what the best dosage is for you.

Don't give up on aspirin too quickly. Different brands may reduce the side effects. However, if you experience any of the allergic symptoms mentioned above, these can be more serious. You should then stop taking aspirin and notify your physician immediately.

Non-Steroidal Anti-Inflammatory Drugs (NSAIDs)

Non-steroidal anti-inflammatory drugs (NSAIDs) were cleverly named because they reduce inflammation, but don't contain steroids! In treating OA they work similarly to aspirin. They relieve pain and they also reduce inflammation. Because they do this, NSAIDs are the primary group of medications used for OA. Although inflammation is a more severe problem for someone who has an inflammatory disease such as rheumatoid arthritis than for someone with OA, it is still beneficial to be able to control any inflammation (however mild) that may occur.

Comparing Aspirin and NSAIDs

Aspirin is actually a type of NSAID. However, it's usually considered separately from the other drugs in this category. How are aspirin and NSAIDs similar? In general, NSAIDs have comparable effects to aspirin in reducing pain and inflammation. They also both work in the same way by blocking the formation of prostaglandins.

However, there are some important differences between aspirin and NSAIDs. Aspirin can be obtained over the counter. On the other hand, most NSAIDs require a doctor's prescription. They usually cost more than aspirin, too. But NSAIDs may be easier to take since you don't have to swallow as many tablets nor do you have to take them as often.

Examples of NSAIDs

There are many different types of NSAIDs. The main difference between them is their chemical molecular structure. (Sorry, further information on this point is slightly beyond the scope of this book!)

Some of the more common NSAIDs are listed below alphabetically. The names given first are the brand names, followed by their generic names in parentheses. Newer NSAIDs are coming out all the time.

- Clinoril (sulindac)
- Dolobid (diflunisal)
- Feldene (piroxicam)
- Indocin (indomethacin)
- Meclomen (meclofenamate)
- Motrin, Rufen (ibuprofen)
- Nalfon (fenoprofen)
- Naprosyn (naproxen)
- Orudis (ketoprofen)
- Tolectin (tolmetin)

These drugs are all available by prescription only. However, there are some from the ibuprofen "family" that are available over the counter. Examples of those are Advil, Medipren, and Nuprin.

Any Problems?

As with aspirin or any of the other medication discussed, NSAIDs do have side effects. Some of the more common ones are stomach pains and cramps, nausea, vomiting, diarrhea, constipation, bleeding from the stomach, and ulcers. Headaches, ringing in the ears, and blurred vision may also occur. Just as certain people may develop aspirin allergies, some may also experience these symptoms when taking NSAIDs. If this occurs, the medication should be stopped and a physician notified immediately.

Analgesics (Painkiller Drugs)

As you well know, painkillers are a major part of OA treatment programs. Other than aspirin and other non-steroidal anti-inflammatories, one of the most widely known examples of painkillers is the acetaminophen family, including such better known names as Tylenol, Datril, or Tempra. They can be very useful in treating OA. Other analgesics that may need to be prescribed for OA include propoxyphene (better known as Darvon or Darvocet), oxycodone (better known as Percodan or Percocet), Vicodin, and Demerol.

There are two main disadvantages to the use of painkillers. First, your body may become used to painkillers fairly quickly. As a result, they become much less effective after a long period of time. You need more of them to produce the same effect. This is known as "tolerance." You may need to continuously increase your dose so that it keeps working, and this can lead to addiction. Your addiction may be psychological as well as physiological! And second, painkillers can have significant side effects, including upset stomach, constipation, and changes in mental state. Most of the side effects merely add to the problems that come with your condition.

Corticosteroids

Corticosteroids (called steroids, for short) have been shown to be effective in treating a number of arthritic diseases. Corticosteroids are hormones that are produced by the cortex of the adrenal glands. Nowadays all corticosteroids used in the treatment of disease are produced synthetically.

Corticosteroids are very effective anti-inflammatory drugs. They can quickly reduce pain, inflammation, allergic reactions, asthma attacks, and colitis attacks. But although they can relieve inflammatory symptoms very effectively, they do not stop the underlying cause of the disease. Most physicians advise against the use of oral steroids for OA because there can be severe side effects.

How Can Steroids Be Helpful?

Since steroids are usually not part of treatment for OA, what's the point of mentioning them? Well, there are times when injecting steroids directly into a joint affected by OA can be helpful. For example, if your knee joint is so painful that you are unable to comply with other aspects of your treatment program (such as exercise) or if you can't walk at all, local injections of steroids may help to improve your mobility and reduce pain. Painful joints may become free of pain for fairly long periods of time. This will allow you to exercise (among other things!). Hopefully, by doing your exercises, your joints will loosen up sufficiently so that you can continue your treatment program without steroids.

There's another advantage to injecting steroids directly into a joint—you won't experience any of the usual side effects seen with oral steroids! But don't get excited now. There are a few problems with steroid injections. The primary problem is the possibility of joint infection where the needle enters the body. If infection is present in or near the joint, injections are not a good idea. Another problem is that repeated injections may cause cartilage damage or destruction. If affected joints are weak or if cartilage destruction is severe, steroid injection is not recommended. If a number of joints are affected by OA, it may be unwise or even impossible to inject each joint. Finally, you may be tempted to overdo it if you feel relief from pain after your injections. Don't give in! Your joint problem is not cured, and you run the risk of causing further damage if you're not careful. Don't let a temporary pain-free feeling affect your long-term problem of coping with OA. So prolonged use of injected steroids is not advised. As a temporary measure, maybe. But as a long-term one . . .

ADDITIONAL MEDICATION 'MINDERS

Once you've begun a medication program, make sure you let your physician know how effective the drugs are in helping you with your condition. Any significant changes in your health, whether good or bad, should be reported to your physician. In this way, your doctor will best be able to decide whether to keep prescribing the medication you're taking.

You may find that dealing with the same drugstore and pharmacist is very comforting. The more time you spend there, the better the pharmacist will get to know you and your specific case. You'll have somebody else looking out for your welfare in addition to your physician!

It is almost impossible for any physician to keep up with all the thousands of different types of prescription drugs on the market. However, this is the pharmacist's specialty. Frequently, pharmacists know even more than physicians as far as what drugs can go together and what drugs interact dangerously. So it can be very helpful for you to develop a good working relationship with your local pharmacist. Not only will your pharmacist be able to tell you about the medication that has been prescribed for you, but he may be able to help you reduce costs. Occasionally, generic products that cost less than their brand-name counterparts may be available. However, in some individuals the generic drug will not work as well as the brand name medication. If you have a good relationship with your pharmacist, you will find it a lot easier to get the medication you need.

What happens if you go into a pharmacy with a prescription and the pharmacist suggests that you substitute another drug (or a generic one) for the medication that was originally prescribed for you? There may be nothing wrong with this, but it would probably be a good idea to consult your physician before making such a substitution.

You may experience certain emotional reactions to taking medication (such as depression or anger). This must be dealt with. (If necessary, look back at the chapters on coping with your emotions.) Remember: If it's really necessary for you to take medication, you might as well let it do what it's supposed to do. Accept it and don't let it bother you.

A FINAL PRESCRIPTION

Research often produces new drugs in the fight against OA. By the time you read this book, there may be additional drugs on the market that are far superior to the ones you've been taking. There is nothing wrong with discussing your medication with your physician, asking if new drugs are on the market. But remember, this doesn't mean that these will necessarily be better for you.

This chapter doesn't include all medications used by people with OA. Instead, it emphasizes the more common ones. But at least this information will help you become more familiar with the ones you may hear about. So if your doctor prescribes something new, ask about it. Then if your new medication makes you feel better, you'll know why!

16

Diet

Food, glorious food! Do you like to eat? It's one of the great pleasures of life. But you might have questions about whether your diet will have to change because of your OA. Or maybe friends and family members have told you that you should change the way you eat.

Is there any particular diet that is most appropriate for OA? The answer is a resounding no! There is no particular diet, food, or supplement that will either help or hurt OA. Of course, it's important that your diet be nutritionally sound and well-balanced. A proper diet ensures that we consume all of the necessary vitamins, minerals, and supplements.

There's one main dietary note to keep in mind. You'll want to lose weight if you are overweight. Why? Added weight can put more pressure on the joints that are already affected. Why are you overweight? Don't blame this on your OA! Your weight may increase or decrease and your appetite may change, but this fluctuation probably has nothing to do with your medical condition. Maybe your weight is fluctuating because of weekend binges! Maybe you've gone to some food orgies! Maybe emotional crises have caused you to overeat. So one of the most important things you can do to help your joints is to eat properly and keep your weight at the proper level.

Because diet is on everybody's mind these days, it becomes a very good subject for quacks. Frequently, you'll hear of miracle remedies involving certain types of dietary modifications that are "destined" to cure your OA symptoms. Unfortunately, no diet has yet been invented that can do any such thing.

The types of diets that have been suggested by quacks include ones based on fish, vitamins, and fresh fruits and laxatives, as well as vegetarian diets, low-fat and high-fat diets, low-protein and high-protein diets, and every other combination that you can imagine. But you know by now that there is no such cure for osteoarthritis.

The moral? Eat healthy, eat in moderation, and enjoy!

17

Rest and Exercise

Two of the most important components of any treatment program for OA are rest and exercise. The proper proportion will be determined by your physician or physical therapist specifically for you, since no two people have the same needs.

Let's discuss these two important factors in more detail.

REST

Rest is an important component of treatment for OA. It is necessary to give your joints and muscles a chance to "recharge their batteries." After resting, you will be able to maintain an alert, active state.

Because you have OA, regularly scheduled rest periods may help to keep you as strong as possible for the remainder of your day. However, if you often feel very tired, this may be your body's way of telling you that you need additional rest periods. So pay attention!

Rest is important. But too much rest can be as dangerous as too little rest. Too much rest may allow your muscles and tendons to become weaker and your joints to get stiffer. If you rest too much, your bones may get even softer. You may feel even more tired. The more rest you get, the more you want. This creates a vicious cycle.

Rest is vital to learning to live with OA, but it must be properly prescribed. There are differing opinions regarding how long your rest periods should be. Some people feel you should schedule several five-to-fifteen-minute rest periods per day. Others feel you should schedule two thirty-to-sixty-minute rest periods each day. There are plenty of other opinions, as well. Your physician will help you to determine which rest periods are most appropriate for you. How? By taking into consideration the severity of your disease, your lifestyle, and other aspects of day-to-day living.

How should you rest? Well, you don't have to lie in bed like a mummy! Just being in a relaxed, comfortable position that places little or no stress on your joints is restful.

EXERCISE

Regular exercise is a very important component of your treatment for OA. Why? The goals of exercise are to build and maintain your muscle tone, support and stabilize your joints, reduce your fatigue, and maintain or increase your mobility. It can also help prevent some of the deformities that occasionally occur from OA, as well as improve any joint deformities that may have already occurred. Don't you wish that exercise could do all this instantly?

You should try to participate in activities that emphasize good muscle tone and do not aggravate your OA. For example, walking or swimming may be better than jogging if OA is affecting your knees or hips. It's also a good idea to have a regular exercise program, rather than exercising whenever "the spirit moves you!"

Muscles also grow stronger and become better toned as a result of exercise. This helps to stabilize and strengthen your joints. Exercise is also essential to keeping your body trim. You'll want to keep your muscles firm, firm, firm—which is better than flab, flab, flab! Exercise can also help your body systems to work efficiently.

But remember that you need a proper balance between rest and exercise. Too much exercise may do more harm than good because it can cause greater pain and inflammation in your joints. A proper balance of rest and exercise can best be determined by your physician or other health therapist. However, only by trial and error can you really discover whether you are exercising or resting in the proper amounts.

Is Exercise Good Only for Your Body?

Exercise is as important for your state of mind as it is for your body. When you exercise, you will feel that you are able to do something. Exercise can build up your self-confidence. Do you no longer feel good about yourself because of your medical condition and the way it has changed your image of your body? Exercise can help. It will restore your confidence in your body. When you see how much your performance has improved as a result of exercise, your self-esteem, also, may grow. Exercise clears your mind, keeps you alert, and helps to control some of the unpleasant emotional reactions that may occur from time to time. Exercise can help control stress, as well as emotions such as depression, anger, fear, and frustration.

Exercise can help you to enjoy deep sleep, so that you'll feel better the next day. And unless you exercise alone, you'll also enjoy some healthy social interactions—always good for the mind (as well as the body)!

Getting Started

Your exercise program will be designed especially for you! (Aren't you lucky?) It will be prepared by your physician, physical therapist, occupational therapist, or any combination of these professionals. Your specific exercise program will depend upon the severity of your OA, the severity of your pain and inflammation, your overall physical condition, the medication you're taking, your day-to-day activities, and the joints that are affected.

If your medical condition has kept you from being active, be prepared for a little frustration. When you first begin to exercise again, *wow*, will you be out of shape! That's not a put-down. Your muscles will need time to regain their strength. So any kind of exercise that you do should be implemented gradually. The longer it's been since you've done any exercising, the slower your return should be. To benefit most from an exercise program, you must do it regularly.

Exercising Caution

Make sure you have your doctor's approval before proceeding. Then start building up your exercise ability gradually. Know your limits and don't do more than your doctor or therapist has prescribed.

You'll want to learn the difference between muscle soreness (which is a normal response to exercise) and increased joint pain (which may either mean that you're overdoing it, or that you're participating in an exercise that's a no-no).

Be careful when you exercise. If you exercise a weak joint, you may run the risk of further damaging the joint. Therefore, although exercise doesn't necessarily have to stop if specific joints are weak, it should focus either on joints that aren't affected or very carefully (and minimally) on joints that are.

It's probably not a good idea to participate in high tension exercises, such as weightlifting or ball squeezing. Nor should you become involved in "jerky" sports such as tennis, bowling, or golf. Not only do these require strength that you may not have, but they may put too much immediate pressure on those joints that you don't want to stress. Jogging is another activity that you may wish to avoid. If OA is causing your knees to become sore or swollen, it makes sense not to jog! It can be very stressful on your knees.

Categories of Exercise

What are you trying to accomplish through exercise? The answer to this question usually determines how to categorize exercises. In other words, exercises can be divided into range of motion, stretching, muscle strengthening, and endurance (or functional) exercises.

Range of Motion

A joint's normal movements (in different directions) fall into the category "range of motion." OA may sometimes reduce the range of motion possible in a particular joint. Exercise attempts to stop that reduction. Just as importantly, it tries to gradually increase the range of motion that is possible. These exercises, therefore, are especially important in treatment for OA.

Range of motion exercises stretch joints in various directions by manipulating the muscles attached to them. Range of motion exercises that are involved in OA may be very helpful in preventing loss of motion, restoring lost movement, and reducing stiffness. Range of motion exercises help you to maintain normal movement in your joints. Finally, range of emotion exercises try to prevent the development of any deformity in the joints.

Strengthening Exercises

Some exercises are important because they build up strength in the muscles and other tissues that support the joints and keep them stable. These exercises also help maintain the strength that you already have.

There are two types of strengthening (or muscle-tightening) exercises that may be helpful to you. Isometric exercises are strengthening exercises that do not involve any movement within the joints. You strongly tighten the muscle but do not move the joint. As a result, strength can be improved without further stressing the joints. Resistive exercises actively move the joint against a resistance, such as a weight, or against other objects. Because there is less chance of straining an already fragile joint, isometric exercises are usually considered safer than resistive exercises.

Positioning or Stretching Exercises

Positioning exercises can be very helpful for someone with OA. Hips, knees, hands, and shoulders are particularly vulnerable to OA. By stretching your body into certain positions, you may be able to help yourself avoid some OA-related deformities. Examples of positioning exercises include reaching a high spot on the door and stretching out on your bed.

You can do stretching exercises to relieve any stiffness or tightness in the muscles and tendons surrounding a joint. If pain immobilizes a joint, the muscles controlling that joint are not doing anything. This disuse will adversely affect the muscle, causing such problems as spasms, cramps, and decreased flexibility. Stretching exercises can help get rid of these problems.

Endurance Exercises

Endurance exercises are also referred to as aerobic exercises. These type of exercises are less beneficial for specific joints, but more helpful for overall fitness. They are usually a good complement to range of motion and strengthening exercises. Examples of exercises for endurance are walking, swimming, and bicycling. Endurance exercises build up heart and lung strength. They can also reduce chronic fatigue and improve overall physical fitness.

Active Versus Passive Exercises

You can also categorize exercises as active or passive. If you're moving your body without anyone else helping you, you're doing active exercises. If you're moving it and someone is helping you, these are assisted active exercises. If you "relax" while a physical therapist, family member, or friend moves your joints (which may happen when you've had a severe flare-up), then you're doing passive exercises.

Guidelines for Exercise Benefits

To be sure that you derive the best benefits from an exercise program, there are certain guidelines you should follow:

- Don't feel that you have to wait until you feel better before starting your exercise program. Starting sooner may even help you to feel better more quickly. But get professional advice and supervision.
- Try to build up a tolerance to exercises slowly. You can improve the way your joints and muscles function by regularly increasing the amount of exercise you do, but do this gradually. Too rapid an increase, or too intense an exercise program, may only increase the pain that you're experiencing. It may also damage the very joint that you want to protect and improve.
- If you experience a lot of pain or inflammation in your joints, exercise must be done with much more caution. Isometric exercises may be helpful. Very gentle range of motion exercises may also be suggested.
- Anticipate minor discomfort from exercising. Remember, you're moving joints that may not want to be moved! Bending a joint and stretching the surrounding muscles, tendons, and ligaments may cause some pain. It's a good idea to push a joint actually a little beyond the level at which pain first occurs. This helps to increase joint mobility. Applying heat before exercising may help to relax tense muscles and reduce pain. But if you experience too much discomfort or pain, or if it lasts for a long time, cut back. It may indicate that you're overdoing!
- Aim to do as much exercise as possible on your own, even though you may initially need the help of either a family member or a physical therapist.
- Don't compare your exercise program to somebody else's. You wouldn't compare your doses or types of medication to somebody else's, would you? (Or should you?)

18

Surgery

Not too many people cherish the thought of "going under the knife." In the past, surgery as an OA treatment technique was rarely considered except as a last resort. But recently, because of advances in surgical technology and its more positive outcomes, surgery has been more frequently considered to treat some cases of OA. So let's discuss surgery, and the way it can affect your lifestyle.

When can surgery be helpful? If other approaches (such as medication, rest, physical therapy, and other preventive measures) fail to alleviate pain or to reduce disability or deformity, then surgery may be considered as an alternative procedure. However, most arthritis experts recommend trying all other treatments before considering surgery. If your OA is so severe that it causes constant excruciating pain or significantly limits your mobility, then surgery may be necessary. It can be a very effective way to return to a more satisfactory, active life. It can relieve pain and restore comfort and mobility to joints affected by OA. It can also be useful in correcting serious deformities.

Surgery is usually an elective procedure. Although you may feel you need it because of pain or disability, it's usually not something that is done on an emergency basis.

WHY SURGERY?

If joint cartilage is worn away as a result of OA, the joints may become painful, stiff, weak, or unstable. If this damage becomes severe, then excruciating pain, loss of function, and deformity may result. Weight-bearing joints may be affected to the point where you have great difficulty walking. If OA seriously affects your upper extremities, you may find that you're barely able to perform even the simplest activities of daily living.

Surgical procedures can currently be used on individuals of virtually any age, although your age and overall physical condition will be evaluated to decide if surgery is desirable for you.

WHY NOT SURGERY?

If surgery can do so much good, why isn't it appropriate for everyone? Unfortunately, OA surgery is not a cure! It may help the symptoms, but it won't eliminate the condition. If your OA affects only one joint or a few joints, surgery may return you to a virtually pain-free existence. Even though surgery can't cure the illness, at least it can significantly relieve many of the problems that come with it.

Surgery can be painful and expensive, and it can require a long recovery period. It also keeps you away from certain activities that you normally enjoy. You may argue, though, that your condition before surgery prevented you from doing these things, anyway.

Another problem with surgery is that it's not always successful, although the success rates have been increasing dramatically. If you have a heart condition or lung disease (or if other problems exist), surgery may be contraindicated, since it may pose a higher risk for you even if the outcome is positive.

TYPES OF SURGERY

In determining what type of surgery is to be done, the orthopedic surgeon must consider several factors, including your condition, which joints are affected, the degree to which your joints have been affected, and your age and lifestyle.

Arthroplasty

An increasingly common surgical procedure for osteoarthritis is arthroplasty. This refers to any surgical procedure that restructures a joint.

There are two types of arthroplasty. In one, parts of a damaged joint surface are removed. A surgical reformation, or shaping, of the joint can help to rebuild damaged joints. In this procedure, the ends of the bone where cartilage has worn away are resurfaced or relined. This eliminates the problem of bone or ligament damage due to cartilage erosion. Arthroplasty may actually create a false joint, where only some of the bone in the joint is removed or the bones are realigned.

There's a problem with this, however. Although a partial restoration may restore some function, pain is still possible. The joint may still prove to be unstable if it's a weight-bearing joint. The trend today seems to be away from these partial resolutions to the problem and toward total joint replacement.

The second type of arthroplasty is joint replacement. In joint replacement surgery, the old joint is removed and replaced by an artificial one (a prosthesis), usually constructed of plastic and metal. This is probably the most dramatic and exciting surgical procedure for OA.

Let's Get Hip

The hip joint is the largest joint in the body. It's also one of the most important weight-bearing joints. A problem in this joint can certainly affect you. The hip joint can become rigid and unusable. The pain may make any kind of movement almost impossible.

Several thousand total hip replacements are done each year. It has gotten to the point where hip replacements are considered almost routine surgery—successful more than 95 percent of the time.

Total joint replacement for the hip is the most frequent (and successful) arthroplasty operation. Successful replacements of knee joints are also increasing significantly. Replacement of certain other joints is becoming successful; research and experimentation continue on surgery that can replace joints in the wrists, ankles, elbows, feet, and toes.

Debridement

A relatively minor procedure to remove bone spurs or other bone fragments in the joint is called debridement. This procedure also removes unhealthy, worn-out cartilage from the joint. Although this procedure can be very effective and can do a great job of reducing (if not eliminating) pain, there's one problem. Results from this procedure are usually not permanent. Eventually, it may have to be repeated.

Arthroscopy

Arthroscopy is a relatively new surgical procedure. It makes use of a small periscope-type instrument (the arthroscope) to look into the joint. The arthroscope, which is a little bit wider than a drinking straw, enables the surgeon to see practically everything that's inside the joint. The arthroscope can be useful in diagnosing problems within a joint or for debridement procedures.

Bits of torn bone or cartilage can be shaved or removed during this procedure. Joints may be cleaned out. Little pieces of bone or cartilage that may be floating freely in the joint fluid can be removed during surgery. Arthroscopy is most commonly used on the knee, but can also be used on the hip and shoulder.

Arthrodesis

Another procedure used is called arthrodesis, or surgical fusion. Two bones may be fused together to stabilize or strengthen a weak joint. Although the bones in this joint will no longer be able to move (because the fusion freezes them rigidly in place), at least the joint will be able to support weight more easily and without pain.

Surgical fusion may be used, for example, at the joint at the base of your thumb. This can help to restore at least some degree of mobility to your hand—mobility that may have been lost due to pain and restrictions.

Arthrodesis may also be done on your spine. If damage from OA causes your vertebrae to become wobbly and unstable, this may threaten your spinal cord and seriously damage (or even paralyze) your body.

Arthrodesis is now used more commonly on the wrist, the fingers, the ankle, the toes, and top vertebrae in the neck. For other joints, joint replacement may be more desirable.

Osteotomy

The osteotomy is a procedure that attempts to correct a deformity in a joint. One of the two bones in the joint is cut and reset in a better alignment. Why is this done? If the cartilage on one bone is worn away more than the other, the result is a bad bone alignment in the joint. After the osteotomy, the bones will be in a better position.

Resection

A resection is another surgical procedure where part of a bone, or all of it, is removed. This is usually done in situations where the removal of the bone or joint will not significantly affect mobility. Resection procedures are often done with the metatarsal joint in the feet when it's too painful or difficult to walk. Resection of the end of the ulna bone in the wrist can help reduce pain and deformity of that joint.

WHAT HAPPENS AFTER SURGERY?

After surgery, it's time for rehabilitation. Your program will include rest, physical therapy, and gradually increasing amounts of activity. You'll need plenty of rest. You'll also need time to get used to assistive devices, such as crutches, canes, or splints, that will support the surgically repaired or replaced joints during this phase. You'll probably learn special exercises so you can regain strength and mobility in whatever joint was involved in surgery. (By the way, exercise rehabilitation is good before surgery, too, to make the after-surgery rehabilitation a bit easier.) Be careful. You don't want to take a chance of damaging the joint that has just been repaired! In all probability, it will take at least a few weeks before you can resume your usual routine. You may want to make arrangements to have somebody help out at home for a while following surgery.

THINGS TO THINK ABOUT

Surgery can result in an abrupt change in your condition. It may be permanent or temporary. But there are certainly some important things to think about.

- Ask yourself a very simple question: "Will the surgery make a big difference in the quality of my lifestyle?" If so, fine. Continue to consider it. But if not, why consider it at all?
- Here's something else to be aware of. Although pain can be relieved and a good degree of mobility may be restored, it doesn't mean that you'll be able to get involved in professional football or other strenuous physical activities! Yes, you'll be able to do more, but there'll be differences between what you can do with artificial joints and what you were able to do with the healthy joints you had before developing OA.
- Get a second opinion. This is always important before deciding whether surgery is the treatment for you.
- Ask your primary physician for recommendations regarding who should perform the surgery. You'll probably want an orthopedic surgeon for joint replacement surgery. If surgery is being done on

your hand, for example, you'll probably want a specialist in hand surgery. Your surgeon should be someone you feel comfortable with and who also has extensive experience in exactly the type of surgery you need.

- Discuss what's involved in the operation and what kind of rehabilitation will follow with your doctor. Find out what you will need to know before, during, and after the procedure. Feel free to ask questions. Remember: Preparation for surgery makes the outcome better (and easier)!
- Prepare yourself for extensive rehabilitation after surgery. You'll probably work with a physical therapist, who will prepare a plan that will help you get back "in the swing." In almost all cases, successful surgery depends not only on the surgery itself, but on the diligence with which you participate in rehabilitation *following* the surgery.

19

Activities

What to do, what to do? Sure you have OA, but what does this mean in terms of the basic activities in your life? What *can* you do and what *can't* you do? Even if you feel wonderful, you'll still want to curtail any vigorous activities. You don't want to put any strain on your joints. In fact, you may not even have the strength!

Each person is different. The kinds of things you did before beginning treatment for OA can influence what you can or want to do now. Your current physical condition is also a determining factor. For example, if you've had joint replacement surgery, you'll want to hold off on most exertions until healing has taken place and your doctor has given you the green light (or even a cautious yellow) to continue. So let's discuss some of the more important types of activities that people participate in.

WORKING

Working can be very important for you. Besides being your source of income (can't overlook that!), working will make you feel as if your life is proceeding as usual. You may be concerned (an understatement!) if your OA threatens the possibility of working. This may interfere with your financial security.

Even though you have OA, you'll probably want to do as much of what you used to as possible. Are you afraid that you'll feel like less of a person if you have to stop working? Work is important. It helps you to feel independent. It gives you a sense of self-fulfillment. It provides more financial strength than not working, of course. And it provides a social life.

Many people question whether they should work. If you want to, and you need to, and you can, then you should! You may have to make some modifications because you don't want to chance putting too much stress on your joints. This would only increase your pain and discomfort, and could cause further damage.

Where to Work

Five basic points may help you when you are thinking about working. First of all, ask yourself if you feel comfortable doing the job. Do you feel physically and emotionally capable? Is it something you want to do? Your condition may have made you more aware of your mortality. As a result, you might decide to start doing something you really want to do! Second, does your employer still want you to work there? Or will a new employer hire you, given your present physical condition? Should you even say anything about it? (More about this in a later chapter.) A third very important matter is whether your colleagues will accept you. This, of course, does not necessarily mean that they will even notice your condition. Fourth, will your condition affect your attendence at work or your punctuality? If so, will this cause any difficulties on the job? A fifth factor that may relate to your choice of employment is the amount of stress involved. Stress is certainly a factor you'll want to minimize. You may decide to change jobs if you recognize that your previous job was too stressful.

Stamina Shortage

OA may cause you to experience fatigue, depression, and adjustment problems. This may affect your work productivity, especially if your treatment has not yet been very helpful. Your work rate may slow down, you may be absent more often, and your value to the company may decrease. You simply may not feel physically able to work. You may get tired easily, and feel that you just don't have the stamina necessary to complete your job satisfactorily. You may need to be off your feet more, or you may have been told not to walk up and down stairs. If your employer is aware of any of these problems, you may be afraid that your job will be in jeopardy.

What can you do? Build up your stamina slowly. Don't expect too much. Pacing yourself is probably the most important thing you can do. Take frequent rest breaks to "recharge your batteries." If you're not sure how much you can do, do what you can and let the amount of pain in your body be your guide.

There's no reason to believe that once medication and other components of your treatment program begin to help, you won't be able to continue working. On the other hand, even if you can't succeed at your old job because of its requirements, you still may be able to succeed at another job that requires less physical exertion.

Bending the Rules

Employers are not required by law to make any special provisions for you because you have OA. You still have to do what you're supposed to do. However, if you're an important employee, your company will probably want to retain your services. You may be able to continue working at a particular job with only a few modifications (such as changing your chair, desk, location, or a few of the activities you used to do). Changing your hours and modifying some of your most strenuous activities may also be helpful.

You may be uncomfortable about approaching your employer to find out if these changes can be made. It may bother you to seek special treatment on your job, but this is something you'll have to do. If you are a valued employee, these changes may be small in comparison to the problems your company would face without you (such as hiring a new employee to replace you).

You may find that you have difficulty with other employees if you receive special treatment. This may not be true at all, but your anticipation or apprehension of this happening may cause problems.

Changing Jobs

Don't stay at a job if it's not right for you. Consider transferring to another one or getting additional training to move into a new job. In some cases, individuals with certain job experiences and backgrounds are unable to work in jobs for which they were trained because of their new condition. For example, Larry, age 59, had been working all his life in construction. But doctors felt he shouldn't continue this type of work because it was too strenuous for him. It put too much pressure on his joints. Larry became very depressed. He didn't know what else he could do. He shut down emotionally in order to avoid facing the prospect of not being able to work. He feared that his age would be an obstacle. He was even afraid that he didn't have the ability to go out and get new training. How do you deal with this situation? One way might be to check with the Office of Vocational Rehabilitation (OVR), a service provided by the government. The Office of Vocational Rehabilitation can be a very important resource in helping you get back to work. You'll find office locations throughout your state. Counselors in these offices will work with you to determine exactly what your aptitude is for different jobs. OVR will then provide you with training and support to help you obtain employment in those fields. In addition, they also provide transportation, counseling, placement, and even equipment (when necessary). If you've been having difficulty getting a new job and are not sure how to proceed, calling your local Office of Vocational Rehabilitation may be an excellent way to begin. If you need help in finding jobs that are appropriate for you, you may want to check with the State Employment Services. These services are available free of charge and have specialists that can help you to find jobs that are suitable for your needs.

Is Working Your Only Option?

What are the advantages of working? Some of the benefits are satisfaction, productivity, money, and pride. But what if you can't work? Or what if you're between jobs? A paying job is not the only type of satisfying work. There are plenty of other meaningful, productive activities that can be done voluntarily. Check with nonprofit organizations, hospitals, schools, senior citizen centers, and the like. They can always use some extra help. You'll feel good about yourself, too. Volunteers can also work with religious, political, or charitable organizations.

What if you just don't want to work? Some individuals with OA are happy about not being able to work. But don't use your condition as an excuse for not working. This may indicate that something else is bothering you. You may want to explore this further.

THERAPEUTIC RECREATION

People with OA may still be able to participate in a number of different types of activity including boating, skating, golf, tennis, and dancing. Whether or not you do depends on your condition. If you try an activity without experiencing pain, swelling, or lasting discomfort, you're probably O.K. On the other hand, there may be times when you feel that your condition keeps you from doing it. However, when your doctor approves of an activity, at least you know that you can try it. It's up to you and your doctor to decide which activities are best for you. Certain joints may be stressed by certain activities and, as a result, those activities should be avoided.

You're probably participating in exercises that you might normally participate in to increase muscle strength and maintain range of motion in your joints. The exercises that are found in normal hobbies and other types of pleasurable activities can actually be extensions of these exercises. This is what falls under the category of therapeutic recreation. The advantage of therapeutic recreation, therefore, is that it not only includes exercise that is important for joint mobility, but also that it is fun!

Why is it so helpful to participate in activities that you enjoy? One reason is that they can improve your ability to take care of yourself. They can also help promote and maintain your participation in the normal activities of daily living. They can certainly enhance your social life and improve your spirits as well.

ACTIVITIES OF DAILY LIVING

Among the things you'll do each day are the normal, routine tasks known as the activities of daily living (ADL). But there's a problem. The pain and reduced mobility of OA may limit these activities. This can be frustrating. Why? Probably because prior to being diagnosed, you may have taken such simple tasks for granted. The way you're feeling now, however, may make you depressed and upset, rather than enthusiastic about trying to conquer the problem.

What if you can't do what you want to do? You may not want to ask for help. You may feel that it takes away some of your dignity. This can make you very uncomfortable. However, the future can be brighter! In a very short period of time, you can reorganize your lifestyle, your house, and your daily activities in a way that can reduce your difficulties and salvage a lot of your dignity.

But first, what ADL difficulties might you have? You may have problems getting dressed or undressed. You may have difficulty with bathroom activities, such as bathing and using the toilet. You may also have problems holding a toothbrush or comb, or washing and drying various parts of your body. Or you may have difficulty turning handles and opening doors. You may have trouble opening jars or holding objects that require fine motor coordination. You may have difficulty eating food or preparing it. You may have difficulty moving, walking, or going up or down the stairs. But don't despair. Not all people with OA experience these problems. (And if you do, doesn't it make sense to see what you can do to improve the situation?)

Modifying your lifestyle or your home is not the same as giving in to OA. Rather, these changes will help you learn how to live most effectively and cope most successfully with your condition.

Easing the Load

Your goal is to make daily living as easy as possible. Why? Other than protecting your joints and relieving pain, one of the most important components of your treatment program for OA is energy conservation. So you'll want to eliminate those activities that aren't necessary and simplify those that are! Conserving your energy can be very important in helping you to reduce stress in your joints. It can also help you to avoid much of the excessive fatigue that can be a negative factor in living with OA.

In many cases, problems with daily living can be conquered without professional help. It can be very satisfying for you to develop your own solutions to these problems. This can be one of the most important ways of coping with OA. Of course, any questions you have can be bounced off physicians, physical therapists, or occupational therapists. In fact, one of the occupational therapist's main goals is to help you solve any problems in daily living, especially those at home or those related to your occupation. This will greatly improve your overall functioning.

Start by trying to evaluate everything you do on a day-to-day basis and seeing how you can make every single thing you do easier. Realistically, you know that you cannot eliminate all of the activities that you need to do around your home. However, what's wrong with finding easier ways of doing them? Is this taking the lazy way out? Of course not. You are simply recognizing that every bit of energy you save from one activity will give you more energy to do something else.

Any specific suggestions? There are lots of things you can do to help yourself with daily living. For example, you may want to reorganize your home and your habits in such a way that makes movement easier and puts things within easy reach. You can replace small handles on drawers with bigger ones. You can lubricate drawers so that they open and close more easily. You can wear clothing that is easier to get on and off. There are a number of different types of gadgets that will make life easier for you.

You'll also want to learn how to moderate your activities. Plan them out carefully and pace yourself. One thing you may find helpful is to chart out your activities, including required activities, as well as social and leisure activities. This may help you to become better organized so that you can pace yourself more effectively.

Try to plan activities in advance so that you can figure out exactly how you're going to do them, what equipment you're going to need, and how much time you can spend doing them in between rest periods. Planning will help you to reduce the amount of strain, both physical and emotional, that you may experience, and will keep you from getting overtired.

Try to reduce the amount of energy you expend in performing any activity. If necessary, modify the method that you use. Try to use any assistance devices or equipment that you can to conserve energy and protect your joints. Eliminate any unnecessary activity. Rest intermittently, frequently, and whenever needed. You'll then be able to do more of what you want or need to do. And you'll accomplish it in a healthier way.

Any activities that cause you pain should be modified as much as possible. If you've already reduced a task to the bare minimum, and absolutely can't do anything more about it, put a limit on how much pain you're going to let yourself endure. In general, you may want to avoid pain that lasts longer than fifteen to twenty minutes.

Support Devices

There are many different types of support and self-help devices that can help you in your daily activities. You can buy or borrow many of them from organizations, hospitals, and volunteer agencies. The three main categories of support devices are the resting devices (which are used when you're not doing anything and are designed to immobilize affected joints), the functional devices (which are used when you're doing something to strengthen or protect joints that need protection), and the corrective devices (which are used when you are inactive, but are designed to strengthen, relieve, or correct a problem).

Any support devices that you purchase or develop should meet certain requirements. They should be durable, lightweight, economical, pleasing to the eye, versatile, and, most importantly, useful!

The support devices that you may find most helpful in daily living can be used in five main ways: (1) bath and toilet aids (such as raised toilet seats, handles, bath or shower seats, and rubber mats); (2) dressing aids (such as clothing with Velcrow fasteners instead of buttons, shoes that are easier to get on, hooks and pull strings for pulling up zippers, etc.); (3) walking aids (such as canes, crutches, walkers, sticks, and other supportive devices); (4) eating aids (such as special long-handled or thick-handled utensils); and (5) household aids (such as book rests, groping tools, and jar openers).

There are many helpful tools and devices available in each category. Going into detail about these devices, however, is beyond the scope of this book. To find out more about specific devices you can use, you may want to consult the Arthritis Foundation or other sources of support. The Arthritis Foundation publishes a self-help manual that includes types of devices, their purchase prices, and resources designed to help solve many of the different problems with daily living. Also, many pharmacies and surgical supply firms have booklets for you to look at before purchasing any device.

Remember that any special devices needed to make your home more "OA-suitable" are tax-deductible because of your condition. Obtain a prescription from your physician for any necessary equipment in case it's necessary when filing your income tax returns.

How do you cope with these support devices? Remember that using a cane, crutch, splint, or any other device is not "giving in" to OA. It's not a sign of weakness. These devices do not lead to "dependency" on them; rather, they allow independence! They speed up activities, permit other activities previously too difficult to do, and help permit joint rest and protection. Does it embarrass you to have to use a cane, splint, or brace? Don't let it. Tell yourself how much it's helping you. Using one of these devices to help your joints is not dissimilar to using glasses to help your eyes! What's more important—support devices and independence, or avoiding "embarrassment" and dependence?

A FINAL EXERTION

Keeping active is a very important part of coping with OA. You want to feel productive and enjoy life. You don't want to let osteoarthritis confine you to your closet. So don't let it. Do what you physically can, but *do*. . . .

20

Financial Problems

Having OA can be a pain in the pocketbook! Any chronic illness can be expensive, and OA is no exception. The cost of having arthritis ranges up to billions of dollars in the United States. However, the cost of living with OA that is the most devastating is the human cost: the pain and suffering that must be endured.

Why are the financial costs so high? The cost of treatment and other medical costs, as well as the cost of medication, physical therapy, and other rehabilitative therapies, all add up. Medical costs build up as a result of doctor's visits, laboratory tests, physical or occupational therapy, drugs, surgery, support devices, transportation, counseling sessions, and homemakers' services. In addition, money is lost because of the number of missed work days resulting from OA. And there are other expenses too. How about the billions of dollars that are spent on quack remedies? The costs (and their sources) vary considerably for each person with OA. It doesn't take long for financial security to drain into a financial problem.

INSURANCE CAN BE AN ASSURANCE

Fortunately, some people can have some of their costs defrayed by insurance. Insurance coverage is essential. For individuals with OA, certain costs may be reimbursed by the insurance company. Insurance companies do cover a number of medical costs. But what happens if you run out of money or insurance, or if your coverage is not good enough? Because you have a chronic illness, you may have more difficulty getting either life or health insurance. Speak to a reputable insurance agent and find out exactly what you are entitled to. Also speak with a social worker to learn what your community offers in the way of aid.

COSTS AT WORK AND AT HOME

What if you can't work, or are only able to hold down a part-time job? Your condition may affect your ability to work. This may cause problems with your job. So it's possible that your "employability" will be reduced because of your OA. Financial problems may arise from lost earnings or income.

Osteoarthritis can also be costly because of changes at home. You may need to have other people help you, or you may need to make renovations in your home. You may need someone to help around the house, such as a cleaning person. All of these things cost money, adding to your financial burden. As your medical costs rise, your budget becomes tighter and tighter. If costs continue to skyrocket, you may feel like you're being strangled!

CAN ANYTHING HELP?

Although OA can be an expensive disease, it need not be alarmingly so if you're careful. If you take proper care of yourself and begin treatment as early as possible, you can prevent more serious (and expensive) problems from arising.

If medical costs are overwhelming you, consider attending a clinic. Because clinics usually operate on a sliding-scale fee schedule, you may be able to get quality medical care at a reduced cost. In some cases, you may even see the same physician you'd normally see, since many physicians graciously donate their time to clinics.

The use of generic medication can save you money. Generic medication is sold by its chemical name rather than by a more common brand name. Ask your physician if it's acceptable to take generic medication. (Remember, not all generics work as well as brand name medication.) You can also save money by refusing to shell out great amounts for quack remedies.

If you are experiencing financial problems, you may want to check with either the Arthritis Foundation or the Department of Social Services. They may be able to provide you with information, resources, and, in some cases, emergency assistance. The Arthritis Foundation can tell you which benefits you may be qualified for and how to apply for them.

So before you do anything, talk to people. Find out what others have done. How do you find them? Ask your physician or nurse for suggestions, or contact your local chapter of the Arthritis Foundation for ideas. Speak to others in similar situations to find out how they handle their money problems. Even though you may initially be embarrassed to bring up the subject, the common bond that exists among people with OA tends to smooth this over rather quickly. You'll be glad you brought it up!

UNCLE SAM TO THE RESCUE

Some government insurance programs may be very important sources of financial support. You may be covered (at least to some degree) by Medicare, where eligibility is determined by age, chronic disability, or both; Medicaid, where benefits vary from state to state; or social security disability insurance. Let's discuss these different government programs, what they do, and how you can participate (if you're eligible).

Social Security (Disability)

If you are unable to work because of your OA, you may be eligible for disability benefits. However, you may experience all kinds of legal problems because of the many different definitions of disability.

The Social Security Disability Program is a federal government program. It is administered and run by the Social Security Administration. The money that funds the Social Security Benefit Plan comes from workers and their employers. Therefore, one of the main requirements for receiving benefits is that you have worked for five out of the ten years prior to your disability. However, if you become disabled before turning thirty-one, the five-year requirement is reduced to one and a half years.

Benefits are available from the Social Security Disability Program to those of you who fit into the following categories:

1. Individuals under the age of 22 who were disabled before that age and are still disabled.
2. Widows who are disabled.
3. Widowers who are disabled and also dependent.

There are also other specific cases that may entitle you to benefits.

There is one very rigid rule that the Social Security Administration enforces in order for benefits to be approved. This guideline is: "The physical or mental impairment must prevent you from doing any substantial, gainful work, and is expected to last (or has lasted) for at least twelve months, or is expected to result in death." In other words, it is expected that your disability prevents you from doing any meaningful work. This must be the case if you are applying for disability benefits.

Once you meet eligibility requirements for disability benefits, does that mean that cash will start pouring in? Not so fast! There are still other steps that you have to go through. You'll have to provide the names and addresses of people involved in treating you, including physicians, hospitals, and clinics. Medical records must be provided, substantiating the dates and treatments prescribed. This information will be evaluated by a Social Security team (including a physician), and additional tests may sometimes be required to support your claim.

Supplemental Security Income (SSI)

Once you apply for Social Security benefits, you also become eligible for Supplemental Security Income. This leads to eligibility for Medicaid. The Supplementary Security Income Program is also run by the Social Security Administration, which operates the Social Security Benefit Program. However, whereas Social Security benefits come from workers and their employers, SSI comes from a general treasury fund.

SSI benefits are available to individuals sixty-five and over, the blind, and the disabled. The requirements for receiving SSI include the same definitions of disability that are used for Social Security benefits.

Medicaid

Medicaid is the more commonly used term for Medical Assistance. Benefits are provided automatically for anyone who qualifies for Supplemental Security Income. Medicaid will cover virtually any medical-related expense, as long as you go to a professional who is a "participating provider." This provider is then directly reimbursed by the state for the service provided to you.

Medicaid applies if you are sixty-five or over and are receiving Social Security, or if you are under sixty-five and have met the Social Security requirements for disability. In addition, Medicaid is provided to families on welfare, and to children under age twenty-one.

Medicare

Medicare is another part of the Social Security Administration. There are two components to the Medicare Program. The medical insurance component helps you to pay for physicians' services and outpatient services, including physical therapy and speech pathology. The hospital insurance component covers inpatient care and nursing care within a facility.

Medicare benefits are limited and rigidly evaluated. They are only applied to charges that are deemed reasonable and necessary in treating your disease. In order to be eligible for Medicare benefits, you must have received disability checks for at least two consecutive years. This applies only if you are under 65, since Medicare benefits are provided to anyone 65 or over.

WHAT SHOULD YOU DO?

To determine whether any of these programs are applicable to you, contact your local Socal Security office. In addition, consult your physician or your local support groups. These sources should provide you with valuable information that will assist you in determining which programs can help you. But beware. These programs are strict. They are more eager (so it seems) to reject your claim than to accept it. You can appeal if your application is rejected, but this becomes even more aggravating. Want some advice? Talk to people who have been through it. Talk with members of your local support groups. Fight for your rights–and for your dollars.

$UMMING UP

Although OA can be costly, there's still some hope. More and more people are learning about its costly impact. Hopefully, the variety of insurance coverages available to you will increase, more provisions will be made for meeting your expenses, and requirements and application procedures will become more humane.

21

Traveling

Gene was a 62-year-old accountant. One reason why he always enjoyed working hard at his job was that it provided him with an income sufficient to take his family on luxurious annual vacations. He and his family would spend many happy weeks in many different parts of the world. However, since he was diagnosed with OA, Gene had not taken any trips at all. Why? You see, Gene was afraid that his pain would interfere with his sightseeing plans, so he didn't want to go at all. Need it be this way? Definitely not. Very few restrictions need to be placed on your travel plans. As a matter of fact, you can probably go just about anywhere!

If you think you might like to travel, discuss it with your physician first. Chances are that if you're able to get around your own neighborhood without assistance, you can probably handle traveling with confidence. If you do have difficulty getting around, you'll want to be more selective about where you go. Some people opt to use wheelchairs to protect their joints, as well as to increase the distance they can travel. Using a wheelchair might not be a bad idea for these people. But others are afraid of being seen in a wheelchair, or are even more afraid that once they use them, they'll be stuck in them forever. Neither of these fears is valid, but both can interfere with happy travel plans. Work on them.

Do all individuals with OA avoid traveling? No. Some don't travel simply because they feel it's too expensive. This may have nothing to do with OA. But plenty of others do travel, whether their trips are short or long. Some travel simply to prove to themselves that they can. This doesn't mean that there are no fears attached. But they do want to prove to themselves that they can do it—that traveling, one of life's pleasures, is possible for them too. As with any other aspect of living with your OA, planning ahead and taking the proper precautions can allow you to travel with a free mind (although not with free airfare!). How should you plan ahead for a vacation? Let's explore some of the things you should do.

When making hotel reservations or other accommodations, make sure that they fit your needs. You'll want to know where you can get proper medical care if necessary. So prepare for this. Write out a list of clinics, hospitals, and physicians in different parts of the world where you may be traveling. In addition, find out if there is a local chapter of the Arthritis Foundation at your destination. This can be very comforting to know.

TAKE MEDICATION AND OTHER SUPPLIES

One of your biggest concerns about traveling may be: What happens if I run out of sufficient medication or other supplies? There are two things you can do. First, have extra medication, equipment, and supplies packed in case any unexpected situations arise. Second, ask your physician to write up extra prescriptions to take with you. At least you'll be prepared if you need more. You may also want to ask if you can keep your doctor "on call," so that you can contact him or her in case there's an emergency. If you're going to a foreign country, you may want the prescription translated into the language of that country in case the pharmacist has difficulty understanding English. If you are flying (in a plane!), you should carry medication and other necessary supplies with you. Do not pack all supplies in your luggage. Why? If your luggage ends up in Des Moines when you're flying to Miami, you don't want to be left without what you need. Besides, if for any reason you need a pill during the flight, it would be rather inconsiderate of you to ask the flight attendant to climb down into the baggage hold to get it!

IDENTIFY YOURSELF!

It's always a good idea to travel with complete identification, not just for your luggage but for yourself. The Medic Alert bracelet is accepted worldwide as identification of a person with a medical problem. In addition, make sure your wallet contains an identification card with complete details about your condition, the type of medication you need, and any other pertinent information. Again, if you're going to a foreign country, you might make sure that this information is translated into the language of that country. What if foreign languages were never your forte? Try checking with a teacher of that particular foreign language in a local school. Check with the airline that travels to that country. Representatives who speak the language would probably be willing to translate for you. As a last resort, you may want to check with the foreign embassy of that particular country. This may take a little extra time, but your mind will be more at ease when you do travel.

AIRPLANE ANTICS

Let's say your vacation is set, you're flying to Paradise, and you're now making final preparations before leaving for the airport. Any special considerations? You bet!

If you have any physical restrictions, discuss these in advance, either with an airline representative or with your travel agent. Airlines frequently have special services for individuals with restricted mobility. For example, you may be able to board early, select your seat in advance, have wheelchair access to and from the gate, and have special meals, if necessary. If you have your own wheelchair and you plan on traveling with it, check with an airline representative to find out what regulations apply.

CRUISES

More and more cruise ships have special accommodations for people with physical restrictions. Some have rooms specifically designed for individuals with limited mobility. Ramps and wide doorways may be available, too. If you're planning on taking a cruise, make sure that you know what ports of call the ship will be stopping at. In certain Caribbean ports, for example, the ship does not dock at the pier. Rather, it drops anchor away from the pier and small boats are used to get you ashore. This may be more difficult for you to handle if you have any physical restrictions. Again, if you're taking your own wheelchair, be sure to find out what regulations may apply.

TRAIN TRAVEL

Quite a variety of passenger trains exists throughout the country and abroad. Some trains are very accessible for individuals with disabilities. Others are not as accommodating. If you're thinking of traveling by train, speak with a railroad representative or your travel agent before making a final decision.

BUS TRAVEL

Bus travel is becoming easier for people with disabilities. Even if you need a wheelchair, it can probably be stowed and somebody can help you get on and off the bus.

A FINAL CONFIRMATION

Remember, not everyone is like Gene. Many individuals with OA feel absolutely no reluctance to travel anywhere. If you haven't traveled recently, you may want to build up your confidence by taking short trips first. Taking a three-month trip around the world might be a bit much! Even an overnight trip might be traumatic. Start with a couple of day trips, then weekend trips, working your way up to short-distance, week-long excursions. Expanding your travel activities slowly is a good way to develop your confidence. There are special travel agencies for people with disabilities. Look in your local Yellow Pages.

A lot of information has been provided here—mostly precautionary, but nevertheless realistic and sensible. You may need extra time to prepare for your vacation (more time than the "average" traveler). However, with this extra preparation you should be able to enjoy a wonderful vacation, just as anybody else would. Don't forget to send me a postcard!

22

Quackery

Edith was frustrated. She had been taking medication for months to relieve her OA pain. Although her pain had somewhat diminished, she still wasn't able to do what she wanted to do. Doctors constantly told her there was nothing else that could be done for her at this point. Therefore, her eyes lit up when she read an advertisement for a "cure" for OA. Without thinking twice, she wrote out a check for $39.95 and mailed it to the "phamaceutical" company that described a particular nutritional supplement which guaranteed it would "relieve your arthritis symptoms in less than thirty days."

Three weeks later she received the small vial of bitter-tasting pills. When she had finished all the pills after thirty days, she not only realized that her physical pain had remained the same (fortunately, she had continued to follow the treatment program prescribed by her physician), but she also had the added mental anguish of knowing that she had been duped!

When you're dealing with something as lasting and uncomfortable as OA, it's important that your illness be treated properly. But what if you become impatient with your treatment? What if it doesn't seem to bring about results as quickly as you'd like? You may become tempted if somebody suggests a particular technique or item that is the "latest medical cure!" This is the lure of "quackery."

WHAT IS QUACKERY?

Quack remedies are treatments that are fraudulent because they do not have a scientific basis. They do not have a sufficient amount of scientific evidence to prove their effectiveness. In other words, there is no reason to believe that they will work and no real evidence that they do! These quack techniques are usually promoted in an extravagant way. Your vulnerability is what's at stake, and whoever is hawking the technique is liable to take advantage of your condition.

Where did the term "quack" come from? In the seventeenth century, the term "quacksalver" was used to describe a charlatan who bragged that certain products had magic curative powers. These phonies didn't know anything about medicine or about their patients. The term "quack" is an abbreviation for quacksalver.

Not all quacks are blatantly cruel people. Some people believe that their techniques work and think that they can actually help you. In some cases, remedies may be advocated even by doctors and it may be hard to differentiate or distinguish these from legitimate treatments. However, you still want to be wary. You don't want to be the unsuccessful guinea pig who eventually learns that such techniques are worthless!

HOW MUCH DOES QUACKERY COST?

Unfortunately, billions of dollars are spent each year on quack remedies and devices. This has become a very serious problem (except for the quack!). And here's another mind-boggler: For every dollar that is spent on legitimate and appropriate scientific treatment for OA, more than twenty-five dollars is spent on quack remedies, phony pain relievers, and inappropriate cures!

WHO'S SUSCEPTIBLE TO QUACKERY?

If you've been experiencing never-ending pain, increasing disability, and problems with (or deformity of) your joints, you may be vulnerable. If you feel that your physician isn't helping you as much as you'd like, you might find yourself susceptible to the promises of a quack.

Don't be ashamed to admit that you've been approached by, or even considered buying from, a quack. Virtually anybody who has been affected by OA has been taken in at least once. (I won't ask if you're one of them—those sheepish grins give me the answer!) Consider yourself lucky, however, if you recognized your mistake early enough and were able to avoid being taken for another ride.

So why do so many people fall victims to quackery? The quack promises a quick, easy cure for a long-term problem. You already know that traditional treatment programs for OA do not work overnight and that you have to adhere strictly to them in order for them to work. In some cases, especially when you're most vulnerable, it's simply too hard to pass up! You may figure, "What do I have to lose?" (A lot!)

HOW CAN QUACKERY HURT YOU?

What will you lose if you try a quack remedy? Besides money, there are a number of things that you may lose. You may also lose patience, confidence, dignity, courage, and, in certain extreme cases, life!

Money can be a problem. Although it may only cost you a few dollars for a book or copper bracelet, it can get more expensive when fraudulent programs of injections or spa treatments are involved. These may cost thousands of dollars. Remember, a quack isn't in business for ego building or gratification. A quack does it for the money!

Quackery may convince you to forego standard medical treatment. If this happens, you won't derive appropriate benefits from whatever medical treatment can be helpful to you. There is also the danger that the quack approach may cause additional damage. This may occur if the quack treatment actually conceals further deterioration of your joints.

Trying a quack approach may be not only financially draining, but also psychologically draining. You may build up your hopes that something is going to work, and when it doesn't, you may feel even worse than you did before. This disillusionment can certainly undermine your courage and determination to live with your condition. Your patience may be sorely tested. You may find it even more difficult to participate in an appropriate treatment program.

It can be terrible to lose your dignity. You may feel that you've been ripped off, or that somebody has taken advantage of you. Your integrity and pride have been damaged. Don't continue to feel this way. Write off what you've done as experience. Accept the fact that you were deceived and move on to more appropriate treatment.

EXAMPLES OF QUACKERY

The different types of quack techniques may be divided into three categories: drugs, diets, and devices. What are some examples of miracle cures with little validity? Consider some of the following:

- Drugs: Indian medicines, vitamin injections, iodine.
- Diets: Immunized "milk," alfalfa seeds, crow meat, gelatin, seaweed, worms, yogurt, mineral waters, fasting, eating only uncooked foods, eating only cooked foods.

- Devices: Copper bracelets, electric belts, magic horse collars, magnetic devices, zinc disks, teeth extractions, mistletoe, polyvinyl clothing, special underwear, sulfur baths, applications of a hot poker, electric shocks, sitting for prolonged periods in abandoned uranium mines.

A Little More Detail, Please?

Many of the quack remedies are based on changes in diet. Keep in mind that extensive research has indicated that other than eating to keep healthy, no diet has either prevented or exacerbated arthritic problems.

Whenever you read of a "diet to cure arthritis," you should be a little skeptical. Why? The key word is "cure." At the present time, OA cannot be cured. In some cases, these diets may be more damaging because they may not provide you with the nutrients or fluids you need for a balanced, healthy diet. Research hasn't shown any indication that a specialized diet can play a role in helping OA. Therefore, you should beware when an individual says that a particular ingredient will make your OA go away.

Venoms are often advocated as ways to cure arthritis. Venoms from animals or insects such as snakes, ants, or bees have been touted as being the miracle cure for OA. What's the danger? What if you're allergic to these venoms? You might experience reactions that are more serious than even OA itself!

Some people believe that wearing copper bracelets can be helpful because the chemical nature of the copper can alleviate a deficiency within the body. The answer to this is simple: If you enjoy wearing a copper bracelet, and you feel it's attractive and adds to your looks, fine. But don't expect it to result in significant changes in your OA.

Certain clinics may also fall under the quack category if they promise miraculous cures costing a mere several thousand dollars. It is true that in these days you get what you pay for. This may cause the unwary individual to believe that paying a lot of money will increase the likelihood of success. Promoters are aware of this, and will milk you as much as they can.

PROTECT YOURSELF

With all of the unproven methods and quack remedies promoted in magazines, in books, and through different individuals, how do you know which are real and which aren't? It's hard to decide if a remedy is really quackery especially if, while using a quack remedy, your pain goes away! But was it the quack remedy that was responsible for this? Or might this have happened anyway due to your regular treatment program, or for another unrelated reason? What if your symptoms return later in full force? If you're convinced that the quack treatment did cause the remission, dependence on it may prove extremely dangerous.

How can you protect yourself from quacks and their remedies? Before trying anything, investigate it carefully. Be suspicious. Be cautious. Speak to your own physician. You should also beware of other individuals who may claim to be physicians and try to convince you that they have a cure for OA. Check with the Arthritis Foundation, the Food and Drug Administration, or the National Institutes of Health.

Sometimes your physician may not be able to tell you whether these cures are valid. In many cases, physicians are so busy that they may not be aware of, or understand, the technique that the quack is trying to push. This may confirm, in your mind, what the quack has been saying all along: that the medical profession disregards the needs of the person with arthritis and doesn't have time to investigate all the possibilities. This may bother you, and may make you more vulnerable to what the quack is saying. Quacks know this. That's why they're using this argument in the first place! Don't let them cause you to doubt your physician. There may still be good reason to reject the idea that the quack is trying to sell you on.

Although some quack remedies may seem harmless, they can still hurt you if they keep you from following an appropriate treatment program for osteoarthritis. Keep that in mind. Try not to let anyone convince you that you should no longer follow an appropriate treatment. If you have questions about whether your doctor is prescribing the treatment that's best for you, it's better to get a second opinion from another physician than from a quack!

BEWARE OF THE "RED FLAGS"!

What should you beware of? Any of the following could be a give-away that the remedy is quackery:

- Beware of any procedure that promises quick, easy relief of pain.
- Beware of any treatment that advocates a special diet or nutritional approach as the answer to osteoarthritis.
- Beware of any secret formulas, devices, or programs that will "cure" osteoarthritis. At the present time, there is no cure for

OA. If any kind of miraculous discovery were made, you would be sure to learn about it in the newspaper, on the evening news, or from some other reputable source.

- Beware of quacks who claim that their cure or remedy is exclusive or secret. You might ask them why honest people would keep their cure a secret when it could help so many people. Or ask them why you didn't hear about it through more appropriate channels! Scientists who are legitimately a part of the medical world do not keep such discoveries exclusive or secret.
- Beware of any technique that has no scientific proof of its safety or effectiveness. Keep in mind that the promoter probably hasn't had any kind of clinical trials to test the method.
- Beware of anything that is advocated in a rag magazine or tabloid, through a mail promotion, or by somebody that you meet in a store or at a meeting.
- Beware of any advertisements that offer testimonials or case histories of individuals who are satisfied with a particular program or approach. If somebody indeed finds an answer to helping people with arthritis, it will not be necessary to advertise.
- Beware of people who claim that they know exactly what you're going through, what symptoms you're experiencing, and then explain how they're going to help cleanse your body of any poisons it may contain.
- Beware of anybody who attacks the standard medical treatment of osteoarthritis or who states that appropriate medical procedures (such as drugs and surgery) are unnecessary because they're damaging and dangerous. Quacks may claim that medical professionals are deliberately withholding treatment approaches that can be more helpful. Some quacks may accuse the medical profession of trying to interfere with attempts to get their remedy approved. Frequently, these attacks will be launched toward the Arthritis Foundation, the Food and Drug Administration, and even the American Medical Association.
- Beware of the efforts of friends and family to persuade you to try a quack approach. Their suggestions may be harder to resist than advice given by strangers. Your family and friends really want you to feel better. They don't like to see you suffer and are eager to find some kind of solution to your problem. This may make *them* ripe and vulnerable to a quack's suggestions, which they'll then pressure you to try. Now not only will you have to resist the

remedy, but you may also have to conquer the guilt that may arise if you don't try their "cure." ("Why won't you try this, dear? Don't you want to help yourself?")

THE FINAL QUACK UP

It's always important to do the best you can to help yourself. You definitely want to feel better, and you want treatment to do the best it can to help you. You don't want to waste time, money, or psychological energy on quack remedies. Always aim to do the best you can to help yourself, but use appropriate means!

PART IV.
Interacting With Other People

23

Coping With Others—An Introduction

You do not live your life alone (unless you're reading this book on a deserted island in the Pacific). You interact with many people every day. So you'll certainly want to be able to deal with any difficulties in interpersonal relationships. For example, what will others think about your OA? How are they going to react? Are they going to ask questions? What kinds of answers will they want to hear and what kinds won't they? These are some of the questions that may bother you. Since you'll probably be with other people during a good part of your waking hours, it makes sense to be aware of how OA can affect these relationships. Obviously, different problems can exist in different relationships. But before we begin discussing each type of relationship specifically, there are a few general points to be made.

DO UNTO OTHERS . . .

When you interact with others, you don't want to become too engrossed in your own feelings. If you disregard the feelings of others, you'll also prevent them from getting close to you. Consider how others feel, just as you'd like them to consider your feelings. What does this mean? You're not the only one who has to cope with OA. Important people in your life are also having a hard time, simply because you mean a lot to them. Remember that. Some people tend to feel that their problems don't affect anyone else. You might think, "How can they feel upset? It's happening to *me*!" But is that fair? Take your family, for example. A problem for you is also a problem for them. Of course, it may be affecting you differently. You may be the one experiencing the restrictions, the physical changes, as well as the apprehensions and anxieties, but your condition still affects those who care about you. They don't like to see you suffer. If you remember this, you'll be better able to cope with these important people and with your condition.

YOU CAN'T CHANGE OTHERS

Do you feel that if you try hard enough you can change the attitudes, feelings, or behaviors of others? It doesn't happen that way. Whether they accept your osteoarthritis or deny that you have any problem at all, you can't change them. You can only change yourself. Spend more time working on yourself, and worry less about others. They may change, but it will more likely be a result of the changes they see in you. Help yourself. Be your own best friend.

LOOK THROUGH THE EYES OF OTHERS

If you have an argument with someone, you may believe that you're right and the other person is wrong. In this case, nothing will be resolved. Take a moment and look at the situation through the eyes of the other person. What does he or she see? What might the other point of view be? Trying to see the other perspective will help you to better understand the problem.

If you look at the problem only through your own eyes, someone else's behavior may drive you crazy. Looking through the eyes of others can help you better understand them and improve your relationship with them. If you try to have a discussion with them, you will also be able to explain how you feel.

PRIDE, YES! REVENGE, NO!

Revenge! There are times when you might think, "I only wish that ____________ could know what it's like to live with OA for an hour, a day, or a week, so that he/she could understand what I've been going through." But you know this isn't realistic, and you can't sit around waiting for it to happen. Besides, afterward you might not be too pleased with yourself for having such vengeful thoughts. So what should you do? Take pride in yourself. Concentrate on doing what's best for *you*. If you have to be a little more self-centered and a little less concerned about what other people think, just accept this as one more way of coping with your condition.

A LITTLE SELFISHNESS IS O.K.

What happens if you're feeling rotten, but others want you to keep doing more and more? In the past, you may have had trouble saying no, because either you'd feel guilty or you wouldn't want to disappoint someone or hurt their feelings. But now you must curtail your generosity because it can hurt you. Frequently, you may have to give the appearance of being selfish. But don't take this negatively. As long as you don't abuse it, this selfishness can be positive for you. Do for yourself; think of yourself. You're Number One, and that's the way it must be. If you take care of yourself, then you will be in the best possible shape to deal with others. The reverse does not hold true. If you are best for others, you may not be best for yourself.

BRING ON THE WORLD

Now that we've started with some general ideas, let's see how OA can affect different relationships you may have with people. Of course, not every chapter will apply to you. You may either read the chapters that are appropriate for you, or read them all to see how different kinds of problems exist in any relationship.

24

Your Family

Blood is thicker than water! Your family can be a critical factor in your successful adjustment to OA. Why? You're probably with your family more than with anyone else. If you get along well with members of your family, you'll have a solid foundation from which to move toward a triumphant adjustment to your condition.

Let's discuss some of the various types of problems that may pop up with different members of your family.

COPING WITH YOUR SPOUSE

Of course, your marriage will be affected by your OA. But this doesn't mean that problems can't be resolved. Through better communication, understanding, and counseling (if necessary), there are very few problems that can't be worked out. Let's discuss some of the ways in which a marriage may be changed by OA.

Social Life Changes

Have you had to cut back on your social activities because of restrictions caused by OA? You may have to curtail some of the activities that you used to enjoy with your spouse. You may not be able to do as much. This change can be hard to bear, especially if you both had active social lives before the onset of your condition. Because your spouse does not have OA, he or she may feel anger, frustration, or helplessness. If your social life is still on hold even after your condition has stabilized, you'll have to ask yourself if this is due to certain fears or apprehensions. If so, refer to other appropriate chapters (such as Chapter 7, "Fear and Anxieties") for suggestions and support.

If Family Responsibilities Must Change...

OA may create the need for temporary or permanent changes in each family member's responsibilities. This can surely be another potential source of friction between you and your spouse, especially when your spouse receives a heavy share of the load. Reassigning chores to different members of the family can be very difficult for all.

Pat, a 52-year-old housewife, used to make lunch for her husband and children each morning. But with OA, she was just too stiff early in the morning, and was no longer able to do this. So she "transferred" this responsibility to her husband. Since he had difficulty boiling water, he wasn't happy about his new assignment. He, in turn, placed added responsibilities on their teenage children. This created even more tension. Despite the fact that Pat's family loved her and was concerned about her health, they were all understandably upset, especially her husband. How can you adjust your routine as smoothly as possible? Make changes gradually. If you are able to afford household help, some of the burden could be lifted. But regardless of whether you have paid help, try to avoid overwhelming your spouse. Be realistic in your expectations.

How else can you help your spouse to adjust to greater burdens? Make sure free time is still available for the pleasures of life. It's only when the new responsibilities seem to be all consuming that serious problems occur. Look at any lifestyle changes through the eyes of your spouse. Consider how you'd feel if the situation were reversed. Think how upsetting it would be if you no longer had time for things you enjoyed because of added responsibilities and pressures. Discuss the problem reasonably, and be gentle.

Denial

What should you do if your spouse doesn't accept that you have OA? You might hear, "Oh, come on, you don't seem to be in that much pain. What are you complaining about?" Your spouse's misconceptions may be tough to swallow. You can try to educate your spouse, but don't go overboard. Constantly badgering about all of the things that have changed because of your OA certainly won't convince someone who has obviously been denying its very existence. Your spouse will not accept your condition until ready to do so. Concentrate on your own feelings. Others' feelings may change, but slowly.

In Sickness and in Health? Sorry!

Unfortunately, some marriages have ended because of chronic illness. The restrictions of OA can drive wedges into what may have previously been good marriages. Former feelings of closeness and intimacy may be replaced by the unwelcome feelings of coldness and distance. Some spouses have so much difficulty accepting changes in appearance and behavior that the "magic" seems to be washed right out of the marriage. But it may not be all your spouse's fault. You may be so apprehensive that you can't enjoy your relationship. Your sensitivity may cause you to be less patient. So marital breakups do occur. But realize that about 50 percent of all marriages end in divorce anyway, even when OA is not involved!

Statistics aside, what do you do if your spouse is frightened and "wants out"? Your spouse's fear, your own condition, and your fears of abandonment all combine to create a horrible package of anxiety, depression, hopelessness, and panic. This package isn't one you can (or should) handle alone and, at this point, you probably won't want to talk to your spouse. You may find communication with your spouse either nonexistent or counterproductive. Get some help. Seeking the aid of a professional or an objective outsider may help to smooth over some of the rough edges. If possible, include your mate. But once again, don't force the issue. It's more important for you, at least, to get some counseling. If your marriage does end, outside support will help you to accept and cope with life without your spouse.

What About Money?

Osteoarthritis can present added money problems, especially for your spouse. If you are the breadwinner, your spouse may fear the unpleasant role of becoming more responsible for financial aspects of family management. If your spouse is the major income producer, pressure from the added costs of treatment and medication may be tough. Both you and your spouse will worry about whether all obligations can be met (and whether they can continue to be met). Money concerns are frequently a major source of friction in any marriage. Your medical bills compound the problem. Sit down, talk it over, and be realistic. Although new strains may arise, these things frequently have a way of working themselves out. Be patient, be communicative, and be positive.

Is Sex Affected?

Another important area in which OA may affect a marital relationship concerns sex. Chapter 28, "Sex and Osteoarthritis," provides more information on this important subject.

A Marital (Con) Summation

Coping with your spouse while you have OA can be extremely difficult and, occasionally, impossible. Any marriage has its ups and downs—problems that have to be worked out. Having OA makes relationships more vulnerable to crises and arguments. Working through OA-related problems requires much more attention to your spouse's feelings and needs. But it's worth it. If problem spots can be smoothed out, your spouse can really be your best ally in helping you adjust to your condition.

COPING WITH CHILDREN

Children (regardless of how old!) need a lot of attention, help, and love from their parents. OA can surely be frustrating for everyone if you're unable to provide as much for them as you'd like. You can't do as much or help them as much. This does not mean that you don't love them or that you're not a good parent. Because each person lives differently with osteoarthritis, there's no way of predicting how much it will affect you physically (or even emotionally). It may be hard to acknowledge your shortcomings as a parent. But think about your children. How hard is it for them to deal with your condition?

Spending Time

One of the hardest parts of coping with children is handling their disappointment when you can't do all that they'd like you to do. You want to be a good parent. But what does that entail? Most parents believe that they must spend lots of time with their children by making themselves available to take the children places and by doing things with them. If they don't do this, parents may feel guilty. But OA can be restrictive and may prevent you from doing a lot of what you'd like to do. How do you solve this dilemma? You (and your children) must face the reality of your condition. You did not choose to have OA. Try to spend "quality" time with your children—special time when you really share feelings and activities. You shouldn't be as concerned about "quantity" time—the number of minutes or hours you spend with them. If your time together is special, then this is much more important than the amount of time you share. Your children will do just fine.

Talking with your children and being open with them will also help them better handle your OA. Children, especially older ones, can read most of what has been written for adults. They can ask questions too!

COPING WITH ADOLESCENTS

Adolescents have special needs. After all, this is the age at which teenagers begin to assert their independence. Look out, world! The future generation is coming! Adolescents want to start moving away from the family setting and its responsibilities. Under normal circumstances, this can create problems in many homes. Your OA can cause even more problems. Why? Because of your condition, your adolescent may have to help out more than usual with daily routines and chores. At the same time, the adolescent wants to do less and be away more. What a bummer!

For example, 17-year-old Laurie feels guilty about not helping out more at home, but feels that giving in is a sign of weakness (heaven forbid!) These mixed emotions cause Laurie a lot of anguish, which of course she doesn't want to discuss with her parents. The need to escape seems even greater. So, dear parent, imagine how helpful it can be for you to be aware of your adolescent's feelings. Take the initiative and offer a reasonable compromise. Just showing that you understand will help. Maybe things won't seem so hopeless to the adolescent, after all.

The Need for Friends

Adolescents are usually less interested in spending time with family members, and more interested in being with friends. Your teenager may be able to better cope with how his or her friends perceive your OA because they don't spend much time at your house. Even if your teenager's friends don't know about your condition, your adolescent may be much more sensitive to the situation. Does this sound strange? Most adolescents want to impress their friends. Somehow, having a parent who has trouble walking doesn't quite "fit the bill." Of course, there are some adolescents who are more mature and open about it. The extent of their love for their parent and a sound family relationship minimize the problem. They may sometimes end relationships with those friends who cannot understand the situation. Unfortunately, this is not often the case.

Another problem for your adolescent is transportation (that means you!). Many adolescents count on their parents to drive them to friends' houses, parties, meetings, and so on. But you may not be available (or able) to chauffeur your teenager around as much. As a result, you may feel guilty because you believe that you're not being a good parent. Your teenager, thinking less of you and more of himself or herself, can become upset or even angry. Your teenager, recognizing this selfishness or feeling like too much of a burden, may also feel guilty. The best thing to do is to talk about it.

Talking to Your Adolescent

Understanding the needs of your adolescent can open the doors to much better communication. However, if you want your discussions to be helpful, treat your adolescent like an adult. This will provide the best response. Think about your adolescent's concerns about your condition. Laurie may be very frightened that her father is never going to get better. However, her father can help by reassuring her that his condition is fine and that he's feeling better. If your adolescent feels comfortable talking to you about your OA, encourage it. But remember to respect the rights of those adolescents who would rather not discuss it.

Finally...

Your adolescent may shoulder more responsibilities because of your condition. This may cause problems, especially if your adolescent tries to deny your condition. Some adolescents will be able to deal effectively with their burdens, but some won't. They may simply be unable to handle the pressure. If your adolescent must assume any additional adult responsibilities or jobs because of your condition, consider that he or she may also be ready to enjoy some more adult privileges and pleasures. How can you require teenagers to fulfill adult responsibilities and then deny them adult privileges? If you're apprehensive about their maturity, keep in mind that if they're old enough to do adult chores, they might enjoy some adult privileges as well (within reason, of course). Adolescents will usually be more willing to help out if they know that they will be treated and trusted in a more grown-up way.

COPING WITH PARENTS

Parents usually have trouble dealing with any illness or condition that their child (even an adult "child") may have. Therefore, if your parents are alive, they're probably having a very hard time dealing with your OA. This makes coping harder for you, too. Why? You don't want your parents to suffer or be upset. You'd probably feel guilty if they were suffering.

If your relationship with your parents is good, then you're among the lucky ones. But what if you normally have difficulty dealing with your parents? Having osteoarthritis doesn't help! How have your parents treated you since your diagnosis? Do they ignore or minimize your condition? Or do they smother you?

The Ignorers

Parents who ignore or play down your OA often do so because they can't deal with it. They can't accept the possibility that it might have something to do with them. How? They may be afraid that they did something contributing to the illness or condition. Or maybe they think you inherited the illness or condition from them.

Even if this is far from the truth, it doesn't eliminate the worry underlying such thoughts. To avoid these unpleasant feelings, they may try to deny that you have osteoarthritis. They might minimize it, hoping that it will go away.

The Smotherers

Parents who smother believe that if you have any kind of problem, they must take care of you. Having osteoarthritis certainly fits this requirement. It doesn't matter what your marital status is, or how old you are. What matters to them is that they are your parents. They are responsible for you and must take care of you. The fact that you can take care of yourself doesn't matter. They'll call frequently, asking how you're doing. They'll want to know what they can do to help. They may come over as often as possible to make sure that you're O.K. Whether or not they come, they'll constantly bombard you with questions about your health and activities. What can you do, short of moving out of town and taking on a new identity?

Remember what we said before? It really helps to see a situation through someone else's eyes! Don't you think this holds true here, too? Look at yourself and your condition through the eyes of your parents. How do you think they feel? What do they see? You don't have to agree with them, but understanding how they feel will help you talk to them. Looking at your condition through their eyes will also help any discussions you may have with them, as you try to explain how you feel. It's fine to let them know that it bothers you when they do certain things. You'll feel great if your discussions are more productive.

What if Talking Doesn't Help?

If you have tried to talk to them and haven't succeeded, at least you've tried. That will help you feel a little better! At least you won't feel as if you should do more to convince them to switch to your way of thinking! What do you do then? Concentrate more on helping yourself feel better, regardless of whether they understand or not. If they're unhappy with you because you seem to be rejecting their well-meant intentions, so be it.

By the way, if you're unhappy with parents who are ignorers, you'd probably love them to smother you for a while. And, if you don't like smothering parents, the thought of being left alone is probably very exciting. There's rarely a perfect solution. No one gets along with everyone all the time. Instead of complaining about your parents' faults, try to look at the positives in their behavior. You'll feel better about doing this, too.

How Much Should I Tell?

You know your parents. You know how they react to things. What would you really like to share with them? Would you like to tell them how you're feeling at a particular time? You probably know how they react to good news and bad news, and how they deal with unpleasantness. How will you handle their reactions? All these factors will help you to decide how much to tell them.

Sometimes, it's easier to talk with one parent rather than the other. You might tell one parent what's bothering you, and let that parent tell the other. For example, your mother may be able to get through to your father better than you can. This will help everybody.

You might wish you could share unpleasant feelings with a parent because of the reassurance it would bring. It's nice to know that you don't have to face something unpleasant alone. However, what if your parents can't readily accept your problems even if they wanted to? It may be more detrimental for you to tell them things that they can't handle. So don't impulsively tell them anything. Think about and analyze the situation. Try to understand what you want to share, and what their reactions may be. It's worth the effort. By spending a little time to figure out what's best, you can help yourself feel a lot better. You'll probably improve your relationship with your parents, as well.

25

Friends and Colleagues

Aside from family, the most important people you'll have to deal with are friends and colleagues. Are there any suggestions for coping with these important people? Of course!

COPING WITH YOUR FRIENDS

What reactions have your friends had about your OA? How many of your friends really know what you're going through? They may have read about it, and at first, they may have thought they knew all about it. But because they weren't physically affected, they might not have been able to really understand what you were experiencing. Some wanted to learn more; some wanted to forget what little they knew.

Some friends may be very supportive—maybe *too* supportive. Other friends may not be supportive enough, something that can bother you even more. Your own mood really determines their reactions. If you don't want them around, if you don't want them close to you, or if you don't want them asking questions, and you let them know this, they will probably respect your wishes. But perhaps they won't be there when you really *do* want them around. It's important for you to strike a balance. You may simply want to explain that your feelings change and to please bear with you. You hope they'll understand the fluctuation of your feelings.

Apprehension Keeps Them Away

Friends may not know what to say to you. What should they ask you? How should they talk to you? Their awkwardness can cause so much tension that they don't even want to be with you. They may be so uneasy that they feel, "Why bother?"

Friends may be afraid to call because they don't know how you're feeling. They don't want to run the risk of stirring up unpleasant feelings in you (or in themselves, if they don't know how to respond). On the other hand, there may be times when friends keep asking you how you're feeling and you'd really like to be left alone. Many friendships are lost or hurt because of misunderstandings. These misunderstandings usually involve uncertainty on the part of you or your friends in approaching each other.

Showing Concern

Can anything be done, or are you going to be a hermit for the rest of your life? Don't despair. There are things you can do to improve the situation. Try to set up ground rules with your friends. Tell them how you feel. If you are the kind of person who likes to be asked how you feel, let your friends know. If you'd rather not be asked, let your friends know that, too. If your feelings fluctuate (sometimes feeling talkative about your condition, but at other times reluctant to even think about it), let your friends know. Your changing feelings may be harder for friends to deal with, so let them know that they can talk to you whenever they really want to. You'll let them know if and when you're having trouble.

Clear up the question marks. If you tell your friends how you feel and what your needs and desires are, fewer unknowns will exist. The uneasiness about what to do or say, which can hurt friendships, will be reduced. Your friends will become more aware of your needs, and will feel closer to you and less afraid.

Changing Plans

Don't you love having to change plans with a friend because you're in so much pain that you can't even move? Probably not. So you can understand how your friends might feel if they were to have restrictions placed on activities. This doesn't have to be so. Good friends, who understand or at least try to understand what you're going through, will probably be able to accept these changes. Others may be less willing to put up with them.

Asking for Help

As you learn to live with OA, do you feel a greater need to call on your friends for help? You may need help cleaning the house, getting places, taking care of errands, or purchasing groceries, among other things. Are you becoming more selfish? No, but it may seem that way to you. The reality is that there are certain things you must take care of. So if you need help, reach out for it. If your friends complain or show resentment, try to talk it over with them. Don't wait until a friendship is destroyed to realize that built-up problems should have been discussed earlier, when the conflict could have been resolved. If you try and nothing helps, remember this: If your friends still don't understand, what kind of friends are they, anyway?

Asking for Help Appropriately!

If you do need help, figure out who to ask and what they should do. If your friend Myrna loves gardening, it would probably be best to ask her for help with the rose bushes. If you know that Emma suffers from "supermarketitis," requiring daily therapeutic visits to the local food emporium, then sending her for groceries shouldn't bother her at all. If Mario has a driving phobia, don't ask him to chauffeur you around. Try to arrange for a proper "fit" when asking for help.

Older friendships also tend to be stronger and more resilient. Such friends will probably be more receptive if you ask for favors. Newer or more casual friends should probably not be burdened as much. Without giving a friendship a chance to become firmly planted on your hook, you may lose your prized fish—a good, solid friendship. Don't come on too strong. You might think, "But can't you see that I need help?" The answer is, "Not necessarily."

Don't feel like you must do everything yourself. There's nothing wrong with reaching out for help. But you'll feel better if you try to evaluate who to ask for what kind of help. (By the way, when you feel up to it, a nice way to show your appreciation is through an unsolicited gift or gesture.)

Losing Friends

What if it just doesn't work out the way you want? For example, what if people you thought were your friends don't call or visit. Some are "turned off" by your condition. Maybe they're afraid it's contagious! Others seem reluctant to make any plans with you, saying, "Let's wait and see how you feel." It's sad, but in some cases it just can't be avoided.

It's not your decision! You may wonder if your friends reacted this way because they couldn't handle seeing you in so much discomfort. Were your friends uncomfortable about being with you? Were your friends unsure of what to say or do? Whatever the reason, you've probably learned a hard, unpleasant lesson. Although you may feel sad, you can't change someone else's feelings. Be reassured that most people who lose friends because of OA do make new ones. You really don't want a friend who is uncomfortable with you. There may be times, unfortunately, when a friend or lover cannot handle your condition and you feel as if you've been rejected. This can be devastating! You may feel not only that you have been rejected, but that you will no longer be able to develop any other meaningful relationships. This is not true. You are still the same person you were before, except for the ways that OA has affected you physically. Keep telling yourself this so you can restore any confidence that may have been shaken by this unfortunate rejection.

Usually, however, if rejection occurs or if a relationship breaks up, it couldn't have been too strong to begin with. Many weak relationships have broken up because of medical problems. A sturdy relationship, even if it has to go through some rough times, will probably end up even stronger than before. Remember, you want a friend who likes you the way you are, OA and all! And there are plenty of wonderful, understanding people out there. So don't give up!

COPING WITH COLLEAGUES

We've discussed some of the problems you may have working if you have OA. If you know you're going to work, what kinds of problems might you encounter? You're going to spend several hours each day in contact with the people you work with. You'll certainly want to feel comfortable around them. Let's discuss some ways in which you might encounter difficulties in getting along with your colleagues.

Employer Acceptance or Harassment?

Let's say that you've been working for a while, but your employer has been expressing his displeasure about curtailed work time. What if an ultimatum is given, stating that if productivity does not improve, you will be discharged? (Polite, aren't I?) This is a potential problem. So what do you do? You do the best you can. If an employer doesn't understand enough about OA to know that you must pace yourself and shows little or no willingness to cooperate, then you're probably better off not continuing employment there. You don't want to look for trouble.

For financial reasons, should you wait until your employment is terminated? This idea has its pros and cons. If you receive unemployment benefits for losing your job, this could ease financial burdens. But if subsequent employers are reluctant to hire you because of the grounds for dismissal, is it worth it? Only you can decide, and you'll probably have to base your decision on your own unique situation. It's a very important question, since your psychological state is so important when you cope with OA. If your employment is aggravating you, then changes may have to be made.

Colleague Conflicts?

There should be little for you to worry about as far as colleagues are concerned. For the most part, if you are comfortable with yourself, others will be too. Hopefully, colleagues will take your OA in stride and won't even think about it. This assumes, of course, that these people know about your condition. But what if you don't want to tell anyone? Unless nosy colleagues ask questions, you may decide not to even bother telling them. Obviously, there is no requirement that you do so.

Would it help to provide your colleagues with some basic information on osteoarthritis? It might, although it may not necessarily improve their attitude toward you or the disease. In addition, reading about something doesn't always lead to acceptance. However, at least you'll feel better knowing that you've tried to help them understand more about OA. If they don't, they don't. Remember: You can't change somebody else. If a colleague (or anybody else, for that matter) can't handle or understand what's going on, that's his or her problem. You can try to educate people about OA, but don't make it your problem. If you've got an employer with an open mind, that's terrific. Don't be as concerned about other people who don't understand what you're going through. Concentrate more on doing the best you can.

Time to Punch Out

Whether you need to work or simply enjoy working, you'll certainly want to minimize any potential occupational problems caused by your condition. Take one day at a time. Don't worry about problems that have not, and may never, occur. If your osteoarthritis does cause a problem, be precise in identifying exactly what it is, so that you can employ the best strategies to resolve it.

26

Your Physician

How do you feel about your physician? (What a question!) Some people see physicians as gods. Others feel that they're rich, unconcerned, cold professionals who don't really want to help. Of course, there are other opinions. What's your feeling? This plays a role in determining how your treatment progresses. You may find that your feelings toward your physician (or physicians in general) have changed since your diagnosis. Some people with OA don't have as much confidence in their physicians, figuring that if their problem had been treated differently, maybe their OA would have been better controlled. It may seem that physicians don't know best, and that you yourself know how you feel better than anyone else. Because of all these feelings, as well as the rising costs of medical care, physicians frequently bear the brunt of much hostility. But physicians *do* want to help.

OFFICE VISITS

Since you have osteoarthritis, you will be "enjoying" fairly regular visits to your physician. These appointments aim to carefully monitor your disease. Visits to your physician will also determine if treatment is proceeding properly.

Depending on your condition, the type of treatment you're receiving, and your physician, there may be different types of examinations during the office visit. Various tests are used to check on your health. Blood tests will probably be done often.

So checkups are important to keep your condition under control. Although some patients deny the possibility of any problems and try to avoid regular checkups, the intelligent person is the one who sees the doctor regularly and as "prescribed."

BEING AFRAID OF YOUR PHYSICIAN

Are you hesitant about speaking to your physician? You might be concerned that your physician will not like the way you're taking care of yourself. You might be afraid your doctor will consider you a complainer who's "crying wolf" and so may not listen to you if an emergency occurs. You might be apprehensive that more aggressive treatment will be necessary, such as medication or joint replacement surgery. Despite these concerns, you do want your physician to do the best for you. So try to be completely open and honest about the way you're feeling and what you're doing.

STICK UP FOR YOUR RIGHTS

People like to believe that their physicians know what they're talking about. This doesn't mean, however, that you must blindly accept everything that's said. For the most part, physicians respect the patient who asks questions. Disagreement doesn't mean that your physician will throw you out or even back down. But if you are unsure of why your doctor suggests something, question it. If you don't like a particular treatment or if it does not seem to be working for you, speak up. Don't hold back. You do have the right to question. In fact, you have the obligation to question. Uncertainty will surely make you feel tense. And relaxation is so important. . . .

GETTING SECOND OPINIONS

Because you may not absolutely agree with everything your physician says, and because no physician knows all, you might want a second opinion. You should always get a second opinion before major surgery (unless it's an emergency procedure). But many people are worried about hurting their physician's feelings. Don't let that stop you. Think logically. Most physicians will accept your desire to get a second opinion. It will either confirm what they feel or point out the need for further discussion. If your physician objects to your getting a second opinion, you should certainly question why. This does not suggest, however, that you should make it a habit of going for second opinions. Nor should you continually shop around for the "ideal" physician. No such person exists.

BEING ABLE TO REACH YOUR PHYSICIAN

Do you know what's really frustrating? How about when you call your physician for whatever reason (whether it's an emergency or not) and have to wait long hours before your call is returned? This may be one of your criteria when searching for a physician. Make sure you feel confident that your physician will promptly return your calls.

After you've lived with OA for a while, you'll better know when you should call and when it's not necessary. Certain symptoms, such as intense pain or unusual, prolonged stiffness, may require you to immediately contact your physician. Other symptoms, such as minor aches and pains, may not have to be reported immediately. Discuss this with your physician. Find out how he or she would feel if you were to call when you were having problems. Ask about the kind of things that should be phoned in. Also ask when would be the best time to call.

YOU'RE NOT "LOCKED IN"

If you are not happy with your physician, you're not under any obligation to continue seeing him or her. Don't continue a relationship unless it's a good one. Don't continue going to a particular physician if you feel you can't ask questions, feel intimidated, or feel as if you can't call when there is a problem. Don't stick with your physician if you don't have confidence in what you're told, whether it's about treatment or medication. Finally, don't continue seeing your physician if you feel that he or she doesn't care about you and doesn't have your best interests at heart.

Your honesty is part of a good professional relationship. If your questions or disagreements hurt the relationship, or if you're afraid of being honest, then this physician may not be the one for you.

You may want to discuss all of this with your doctor before making any moves. You might be able to straighten things out and improve the relationship. But if you can't, remember that you're looking out for your health. You want the support of a physician who can meet most of your needs.

27

Comments From Others

As Ralph Kramden of *The Honeymooners* would say, "Some people have a *B-I-G MOUTH!*" You may agree with this when you think of some of the comments you hear from people around you. They may know you have osteoarthritis, but that doesn't mean they know how to talk to you about it or what to say. They may say things that they feel are right, witty, intelligent, or even sympathetic. But you may think otherwise! There are times when a certain comment might make you want to implant your knuckles into the speaker's teeth! Or when a comment might make you wonder if you're talking to a graduate of the Ignoramus School of Tactlessness.

But why are you reading all this? As you know by now, you cannot change other people. You cannot improve their lack of sensitivity or the way they talk. What you *can* do is learn to cope with some of the ridiculous comments that you may hear.

ARE OTHERS BEING CRUEL?

Most people will say things out of sincere concern for you. They may be trying to make you feel better, show their support, or show their interest in you by asking how you feel. Does that mean you must always be receptive to their questions and respond to all of them seriously? It would be nice. The problem is that hearing the same questions over and over can begin to get on your nerves. Initially, you may try to either gently respond to comments and questions or politely change the subject. However, these tactics don't always work. Some people avoid these annoying questions by simply not telling anyone about their condition. However, if your OA is noticeable, certain comments may be directed toward you anyway.

For the purpose of this chapter, let's assume that we're discussing those comments that you can't avoid, from people who haven't yet learned to tune into your feelings. If you haven't heard these, that's great! But read on anyway. You never know when what you read might come in handy!

THREE WAYS OF RESPONDING

Many of the things that people say to you may be legitimate comments, but may bug you just the same. Others may not even deserve answers. Still others may be said without considering your feelings. But it doesn't matter why the comment is inappropriate. What really matters is that you handle these comments in a way that is comfortable for you. There are three ways that this can be done.

The first way is by ignoring the comments. This is not always easy, especially if the person is waiting for your response or seems genuinely insulted by your lack of response. How do you get them to stop asking (short of buying a muzzle!)? Change the subject or walk away—ignore the question.

The second way is by trying to answer their questions in a rational and intelligent way, explaining your answer, how you feel, or whatever it is that you sincerely want to communicate to the other person. But now you may feel like you're banging your head against a wall. What if you just can't convince the other person of what you're trying to say? Such frustration can be painful! There's a limit to how many times you can try to explain something clearly and not have it understood or accepted before you explode. (And this isn't good for your physical health, either!)

What if the first two ways don't do the trick? There's got to be a better way, and there is. The third way is to respond humorously. When should you react this way? If someone says something unreasonable to you or asks you a foolish question that can't really be answered logically, you'll accomplish very little by ignoring it or by trying to reasonably explain your feelings. You don't know if your answer will be accepted or if the interrogation will continue. So, in many cases, the third option, called "paradoxical intention," may be best. The idea behind it is that the person is asking or saying something that is really unanswerable. So you're going to have a little fun with your response. Let's see how it works.

Handling the "Big Mouth" Syndrome

What might you hear? And how should you handle it? Remember, the best response is one that will educate the "commenter." You'd like to explain your situation nicely, in a nonoffensive, sincere way. But you're only human. So how can you respond when you get fed up? Read on . . .

"You Look Awful!"

It can be very upsetting when somebody says, "Wow, you look lousy!" You may feel lousy, but you certainly don't want to be reminded of it. You surely don't want to think that the way you feel is so obvious to others. You'd like to believe that you at least look O.K. to those around you. Even if it's said sympathetically, being told that you don't look well may be insulting. So what do you say? You might respond, "Thank you, so do you!" Or, "Yes, I know. I've worked hard to look that way." Or if you're really in a cynical mood, you might say, "I know I look lousy. That comes from hearing people tell me this!" Of course, you could always say, "That makes sense, since I don't feel so hot, either!"

"Why Do Your Fingers Look Like That?"

Most considerate people won't ask ridiculous questions such as this. But every now and then, you might encounter someone who is so absorbed with himself or herself that common courtesy is overlooked and curiosity takes over. So what do you do if you don't want to explain how the inflammation of OA has affected your joints? You might say, "My fingers did too much walking through the Yellow Pages." Or, "They work better when they look this way!" Or, "My real name is Pinocchio, but it isn't my nose that grows." Of course, you could put the other person on the spot by asking, "What's wrong with them?" as you smile innocently!

Remember: For this approach to work best, you want to respond in a lighthearted way. This will show the person making the comment that you're fine, but you just don't appreciate what he or she is saying.

"Are You Sure You Needed Joint Replacement Surgery?"

What if a friend finds out that you've had a hip replaced and says, "You should have gotten a second opinion. You probably didn't need it." Besides retorting that you did get a second opinion, how else can you respond to this? You might answer by saying, "You're right, I don't need it. I just love being confined to bed!" Or else, "You're right, I should have gone to more doctors. The smell of the antiseptic excites me!" Or, "I decided that I needed it so my leg would be strong enough to kick you in the *#@"#"!"

"What Did You Do to Yourself?"

Some people are convinced that whenever something goes wrong, it is a result of personal neglect. You meet a friend in the street who says, "If only you had eaten better, this wouldn't have happened." You could reply, "What should I eat now, a new joint?" If someone asks why you seem tired, you might respond, "Normally I don't seem so tired, but I just finished a marathon dance contest." Or you could say, "I'm tired from kicking people who keep asking me what I did to myself!" This does not suggest that you be unfeeling in your answers. However, if you need to let the "commenter" know that you don't appreciate these questions, that'll do it!

"How Can You Stand So Much Pain?"

In response to this profoundly sympathetic expression of curiosity, you might want to ask, "What pain? The pain from my joints or the pain I get from these dumb questions!" Or you might want to point out other feelings, such as, "I've grown rather accustomed to not being able to move!" Or you might simply say, "I don't stand it. I usually have to lie down!" People will get the message. You may not like the pain of OA, but at least you're learning to cope with it.

"What's Osteoarthritis?"

Plenty of people are aware of what arthritis is, even if they don't know that what you've got is called osteoarthritis. But how do you respond if somebody asks what it is, or says, "I never heard of OA," and you're tired of explaining? You might say, "Let's forget you even brought it up. Then you can keep your streak going!" Or you could say, "I never heard of it either. How's the weather?" Don't forget: You really don't want to hurt the person's feelings by being sarcastic. However, coping with comments from others can be one of the hardest things about living with OA. There are times when being gentle and tactful with others is less important than helping yourself to handle comments without becoming aggravated.

If the person asks why you sound sarcastic, you can explain that you're not trying to be that way. But the comment you just heard was so ridiculous that you figured the person was trying to be funny. So you decided to have some fun, too! But if the person really wants to know how you feel . . .

You won't always have to use this technique, but you may want to. You'll always come across someone who will say or ask something ridiculous. However, as you learn to feel better about your responses to comments, you'll find that you can handle them more calmly. You won't have to use sarcastic-type comments, and you'll have more fun with humorous, enjoyable ones. You'll keep people on your "friend" list, rather than on your "you know what" list.

What if you're thinking, "I could *never* say those things. It's just not my style." Well, you don't always have to. But you can at least *think* these comments. Even that will help you to feel better!

OTHER LOVABLE COMMENTS

What are some of the other comments that you may hear? How many of these have come your way?—Is osteoarthritis contagious? . . . How do you get dressed? . . . Why don't you quit your job? . . . You should exercise more! . . . Are you sure you can walk up those stairs? . . . Your hands look strange! . . . Rest. Don't do anything! . . . What did the doctor say? . . . How's your hip? . . . What is the prognosis? . . . Wow, have you changed! . . . You must miss the way it was! . . . What's the matter with you? . . . Can I help you? . . . I certainly don't envy you! . . . Your having osteoarthritis is the worst thing I ever heard!

IS THAT ALL?

Volumes would be needed to include all of the comments that you might hear from well-meaning friends or relatives. By reading these examples, you can at least get an idea of how to respond in a humorous way. Look over this list. Can you come up with some goodies? You don't want to be cynical or cruel. Rather, you want to show the speaker that you're feeling well enough to respond lightheartedly.

A FINAL COMMENT

One of the most common and yet most irritating comments that you may hear has been saved for last. Imagine that somebody, who is supposedly sympathetic and trying to help you feel better, turns to you with eyes full of compassion and concern, and says, "I heard about someone who was crippled from osteoarthritis!" As you turn to walk away, you respond, "I heard about someone who was crippled after telling someone with OA what you just told me!" You walk away, head held high and a smile on your face, leaving the astonished well-wisher behind you.

28

Sex and Osteoarthritis

This chapter is *not* rated R, for Restricted. Rather, it is rated E, for Essential. Why? If you are sexually active, living with osteoarthritis can certainly have an impact on your sex life.

Has OA decreased your sexual appetite or ability? This can have an important bearing on the closeness of the relationship with your partner. What kind of sexual relationship did you have before you were diagnosed? (I'm not being nosy. You don't have to write and tell me!) Was it a solid one, or was it on shaky ground? If you had a good sexual relationship, you'll have an easier time getting over any obstacles that OA may have thrown into your sex life. If your sexual relationship wasn't good, it is unlikely that having OA will make it better. You may need some professional help to keep things from breaking down altogether. But don't lose hope. If you unite with your partner to work things out together by reassuring each other, relearning how to please each other, and showing a desire for each other, progress can certainly be made.

WHERE'S THE PROBLEM?

Let's talk about what the problems might be. There can be both physiological and psychological reasons for changes in your sexual appetite. Physiological problems are better suited to specific treatments. Psychological problems are harder to deal with (ah, there's the rub). Let's explore some of the different possibilities.

The Body Beautiful? (Physical Problems)

Can physical problems alter your interest in sex? You bet your hormones they can!

There is no question that OA can have an effect on your sex life. What can cause some of the difficulties? How about pain, stiffness, and fatigue? It's very hard to enjoy sexual activities or even engage in them at all if you're in a lot of pain, or if sex itself becomes painful. Most sexual problems are mechanical, related to pain and joint restrictions, since the genitals are not directly affected by osteoarthritic problems. Many people with OA experience pain in the hip, the knee, or both. These parts of the body can be an important part of sexual activity. Since movement can increase pain, you'll want to minimize your movement or try positions that require less activity on your part.

Because painful movement or restriction of joints can make sex difficult, it's important to explore possible ways of changing this. Try procedures that can help relax your muscles or reduce pain, such as moist heat, warm baths, or compresses. Limbering-up exercises may pave the way to more pleasurable sexual encounters. (This gives new meaning to the term "warm-up," doesn't it?)

Since sexual activity often takes place at night, aspirin (or other painkilling medication) may be taken before the sexual act so that pain relief is at its maximum.

You may want to try different positions. Some of them may put less of a strain on painful or restricted joints. If sexual activity is painful, you may be better off taking a more passive role in your encounters. Assume a less active position. On occasion, the use of simple devices such as pillows or knee pads can make sex a lot less painful.

Is there any particular time of day when you experience less pain? For some people, it may be too uncomfortable to have sex late at night. Others may be too stiff in the morning or the early part of the day. Working these problems out takes the cooperation of both partners. Kids, work, and other responsibilities may interfere, of course, but it's better to have sex at planned times than not at all. Frequently, sexual problems can be helped by using your imagination and experimenting with different varieties (in position, timing, and technique).

Other physical problems can affect both men and women. For example, fatigue can be a factor. If you're tired, you're going to be less interested in sexual activity. This can be a real headache! (Sorry about that!) But if you're uncomfortable or fatigued, hanky-panky will just have to be put on hold. Is this a poor choice of words?

Actually, it may be an excellent idea. After all, just holding each other can be a wonderful experience, too!

What about drugs? Sexual problems may be caused by such medication as painkillers, sedatives, and tranquilizers, or by other types of "drugs" like alcohol. It's true that small amounts of any of these may make you feel more relaxed (increasing the possibility of sex), but too much can work against you. The use of alcohol is notorious in reducing sexual abilities because of its effect on the body.

Some drugs can have a direct effect on sexual desire. For example, certain medication (such as tranquilizers, which reduce your anxiety) can suppress sexual desire or your ability to achieve orgasm. Antihypertensive medication may also have an effect on sexual performance.

What about sex after joint replacement (or other) surgery? Sexual relationships can, in many cases, be resumed once healing has taken place. Many doctors recommend waiting at least six to eight weeks after surgery before resuming intercourse. So make sure you consult your surgeon before resuming sexual activity.

The return to sex can be either extremely pleasurable or extremely disappointing, depending on each participant's point of view. If you were looking for skyrockets, but were very nervous, you may have been disappointed. Inability to perform is not unusual following surgery, but this need not be permanent.

Going Out of Your Head? (Psychological Problems)

Your body isn't the only thing that may affect your sexual interest. Your mind also comes into the picture.

What's the most important sex organ? Think hard now. The correct response is your brain! (Did I catch you?) If a sexual problem exists that is not physiological, then it doesn't exist in your body, but in your mind.

Many people with OA experience a decreased interest in sex. This doesn't necessarily mean that there's something wrong with them. As a matter of fact, decreased sexual interest is common in many chronic illnesses.

Self (and Body) Image

Living with OA may affect your self-esteem. Do you like yourself less because of your condition? If you feel this way, you may be more fearful of rejection by your partner. As a result, you may reduce sexual activity simply to minimize the chances of rejection.

Because self-esteem is a necessary factor in enjoying sexual intimacy, you'll want to improve your ability to like yourself. Feeling good about yourself and your body are very important if you want to enjoy your sexual relationships. It will also make your partner feel more comfortable. On the other hand, if you don't feel good about yourself, this will also affect your partner. This can certainly interfere with closeness!

Your perception of your body can greatly affect your self-esteem. Loss of satisfaction with your own body can decrease your self-esteem. You may feel reluctant to share your body with your spouse or partner. Do you see your body in a distorted way? Alice, a 47-year-old woman married for twenty years, was upset that her condition had resulted in a few joint deformities. She feared that her husband would not want her to touch him because of the way her hands looked. Do you fear that your partner may be less interested in sex because of the way you look? Actually, your partner may not feel this way. But you may try to avoid sex anyway, rather than risk rejection.

Self-consciousness can be a big problem. Some people with OA feel less feminine or masculine because of changes in the way they move or look. How has your condition affected your perception of your sexuality? If having OA makes you feel less sexually attractive (and interestingly, this is not uncommon), then you've targeted an important area to work on. See what things you can change (consider getting advice about clothes, make-up, and other "appearance enhancers"). Try to remember that nobody's perfect. Everybody has flaws. It makes sense to work on enhancing your looks in whatever ways are appropriate. If you are overweight, wear fashions that will trim down your appearance. If you have a big nose, apply make-up so as to give the illusion of a slimmer one. Whatever the problem, there is usually a way to correct it. But improving your mental attitude is just as important. For those problems that can't be modified, use some of the thought-changing procedures described earlier in Chapters 6, 8, and 9. They may be the key to your future happiness!

Emotional Interference

Emotions can get in the way, too! Sexual activity may be restricted because of depression. You may be so withdrawn that you simply have no interest in it. Your anxiety concerning sex itself, the intimacy of your relationship, or your sexual performance can also hold you back. You may be afraid that you just can't "make it."

Any of these can happen to anyone—not just to people with OA. Fortunately, they can also be changed with proper awareness, interaction, improved communication, and therapy (if necessary).

Sexual problems can be frustrating, especially if you don't have a partner. It may be uncomfortable for you to even think about finding someone new, knowing the problems you're having with OA. Take things one step at a time. Be more social, look to make new friends, and try not to worry about the more intimate activities that might occur in the future.

TALK IT OVER

A very important part of sexual relationships is communication. If you and your partner can share thoughts and feelings, you'll be in much better shape to work out any sexual problems that may occur as a result of your condition. If communication problems exist, however, difficulties may be very hard to resolve.

It is important to discuss sexual problems with your partner. Theresa, a 58-year-old housewife, had OA. Her husband Mike felt incapable as her lover because he was unable to get Theresa excited, and because he caused her pain whenever he attempted to make love to her. But Mike may be reassured that these problems could result from OA rather than his inadequacy as a lover. If that's the case, then both Theresa and Mike should explore different methods of igniting sexual flames. Otherwise, unpleasant feelings may develop between them. You can work through such feelings, however. Acknowledge the problem and discuss it with your partner. It can be very helpful to discuss any problems with your physician or other health professionals as well. In many cases, the major problem is that you keep these feelings inside, avoid discussing them, and cause your sex life to dwindle down to nothing.

All that has been said, of course, assumes that your interest in sex is affected by your condition, and that your partner is suffering. But what if the opposite is true? What if you still have normal sexual desires, but your partner is the one who's afraid? Maybe your lover fears hurting you or creating additional problems. Or maybe you're regarded as a fragile flower, easily broken, and your partner is reluctant to be sexually spontaneous. This must be carefully discussed. If one-on-one attempts at working things out don't help, don't hesitate to get some professional assistance. It's well worth it.

A PREGNANT PAUSE

For many people, discussions about sex include the topic of pregnancy. However, many people with OA develop the disease after child-bearing years have passed. Is pregnancy a concern for you? If so, let's address a few points. (If not, you may certainly skip to the next section!). Maybe you're afraid of getting pregnant. These fears can certainly interfere with sexual performance. Even if you use a contraceptive, you may still be nervous, and this may make it hard for you to enjoy sex spontaneously. But sex does not have to be spontaneous in order to be pleasurable. And perhaps there are additional things you can do to decrease your chances of pregnancy. Discuss these with your physician before moving into separate bedrooms!

Should You Conceive?

There are plenty of question marks. What about your medication? What about selfishness or guilt feelings? Will you really be able to care for the baby if your OA is so bad that you can't hold, diaper, or feed the little one? What about breastfeeding? Will your medication enter the breast milk and, in turn, the baby?

Will you have more difficulty conceiving because of OA? No (unless the pain and restricted mobility of your condition prevent you from having intercourse!). Remember, though, that some women have problems conceiving regardless of their medical condition.

Are you afraid that osteoarthritis may cause a difficult or unsafe pregnancy? It shouldn't. OA should not have any effect on your pregnancy. But other problems that can disrupt any normal pregnancy can still occur. Such pleasures as morning sickness, nausea, and fatigue are still possible. Thrilling, right?

The best thing to do is to bring all issues out into the open and discuss them husband and wife, doctor and family, and perhaps obstetrician and rheumatologist. Everyone must get involved in the discussion. We're not dealing with simple questions such as, "Should I take two aspirin today or one?"! We're talking about major considerations that have significant psychological overtones, too.

If You Do Conceive

Pregnancy can place additional stress on you, although it is impossible to predict what will happen during anyone's pregnancy. Pregnancy shouldn't have any major long-range effects on your OA, either beneficial or harmful. As a result, you'll probably decide to attempt (or avoid) pregnancy for the same reasons that others would under non-OA circumstances.

In general, it's usually a good idea to avoid most medication during pregnancy. But this is not always possible. Aspirin, for example, has been used by many women during their pregnancies, without any damage to the fetus. Make sure you check with your physician if you have any questions.

In all cases, don't take decisions regarding medication and pregnancy lightly. And, even more important, don't take decisions into your own hands. That's what you have a doctor for, right?

If OA is affecting your hips, you should take this into consideration when preparing for childbirth. A caesarian section may be necessary if you are unable to get into birth positions.

Remember that in most cases, pregnancy should not be a problem at all, especially if you have only a mild case of OA. What are the keys to a successful pregnancy? Awareness, supervision, and careful planning. Take all these factors into consideration, and then—good luck!

AND NOW THE CLIMAX

Because sex is such an intimate and important part of a marriage (or any serious relationship), the whole relationship can be affected when either or both partners feel there is trouble. Try to discuss this. If necessary, include your physician in a discussion to clarify issues that may not be readily accepted. You can still have a warm relationship even if your sex life is less active, but not if there are bitter feelings and misgivings at the same time. Understanding each other's feelings is a very important part of coping with OA.

Remember: Having OA doesn't mean that sexual activity must be reduced, curtailed, or totally eliminated! As a matter of fact, it can still be as pleasurable and as important as the partners want it to be. (By the way, as long as we're talking about the climax, are you aware that orgasm triggers a release of naturally produced painkillers? What a pleasurable way to reduce pain!)

29

Living With Someone With Osteoarthritis

Illness can create changes in relationships. No kidding! If you live with someone who has OA, you may have a number of concerns. You may now see that person differently. Maybe you are reminded of your own vulnerability. Maybe you had been dependent on that person, and now you have to shoulder more of the burden. What does all this mean? Although you share the concerns of the individual who has osteoarthritis, you also worry about yourself. If you have difficulty dealing with your loved one because of OA, you're not alone. Often, illness in a loved one creates a lot of ambivalent feelings in yourself. Concerns about the future, your loved one's health, and money may be troublesome to you. This is not unusual.

What if you feel anger toward this person, not because of anything that was done, but because of the fact that OA has created changes? This is normal, but may still produce guilt. Why? Because this anger is directed toward somebody who, at the present time, is vulnerable and unable to defend himself or herself.

WHAT CAN YOU DO?

If you are close to someone with OA, you have an important job on your hands. This job is made up of many components, the most important of which is the need to be understanding and supportive. This is very important, whether you live in the same house as the person or are simply a relative or friend. People with OA do not have it easy, but they'll have a much harder time if they feel alone and isolated.

Learn About OA

A great way for you to help is by learning as much as you possibly can about osteoarthritis and its treatment. Do you enjoy worrying? You may have unnecessary worries if you don't know things about OA treatment that the person does. By understanding the treatment program, you can better provide support and understanding.

Know When to Let Go

Don't stay on top of the person. Sure, you'll want to help. But give him or her enough space to regain some control over his or her own life.

How about doctor's visits? If your loved one agrees, you may want to go along for the ride. There may be times when the doctor might want to discuss something with you. It might be a good idea for four ears rather than two ears to listen when the doctor is explaining OA, medication, or other aspects of the treatment program. However, if the person wants to go alone and feels strongly about it, don't force the issue.

Encourage, Don't Pester

Encourage adherence to proper management routines and medication needs. But don't badger. If your loved one is not taking proper care of himself or herself, there is a limit to how much you can do to change things. Screaming usually doesn't help (and it can hurt your vocal cords!). Should you tell the physician if the person is not taking care of himself or herself? That's a hard question to answer. You don't want to overstep your bounds and be resented. At the same time, you don't want to sit back and watch unnecessary problems develop. This is especially true if the person doesn't seem to care. What do you do if he or she just "gives up"? Play each situation by ear. Before deciding whether to say anything, you should discuss it with your loved one. Voice your concerns; mention that you're afraid of a problem becoming worse. Listen to the responses before deciding whether to carry it any further.

Sympathize, Don't Pity

Because of the difficulties that accompany OA and its treatment, you may sympathize with the person. You may feel sad about what he or she has to go through. This may help you to provide beneficial support. But don't go overboard on pity. This can be destructive.

There will be times when the person is so fatigued that little or nothing can be done. At such times, it is not appropriate for you to insist that the person "get up and do something." That won't make him or her feel better! Try to help out. Try to reduce the person's pressures at that time. See if you can take over any of his or her obligations or responsibilities to ease the person's load.

At the same time, don't allow your loved one to baby himself or herself. In general, if the person can do something (even if it takes time), let him or her do it. If you feel that this individual is "copping out" or malingering, both of you should discuss this behavior. Try to make life as normal as possible.

Don't Be Extreme

Frequently, friends or relatives go from one extreme to the other. What does this mean? If the person gets tired, you'll help out. But if the person is no longer tired, will you allow him or her to do what is desired? When feeling better and able to do things, the last thing the person wants is to be told to get into bed and rest. Have faith in your special someone. If the person really doesn't feel well, he or she will rest. Otherwise, let up!

How to Respond

Can you always be sure of your best response? You may feel that at certain times, the best way to respond is with sympathy and understanding. At other times, the best thing may be to just ignore what's going on and walk away. There may be times when you want to joke about OA. But there's no way for you to know for sure. You can't predict the person's needs. How can you help? Lay ground rules. Hopefully, your loved one will initiate this. If not, maybe you can start the discussion. Mention your concerns. Talk about your interest in being as helpful as you possibly can, and ask what you can do to help. Things will move more smoothly if you have a good idea of what to do and when to do it. Even if there are no clear-cut, definite answers, at least there will be some constructive communication. You'll be better able to handle future problems.

Keep Talking

It is very important to have open lines of communication between you and your special someone. This is really the only way you can become aware of his or her physical and emotional condition. If you do listen to your loved one, you can truly help. This doesn't mean that the conversations will always be pleasant. Talking about problems, depression, fears, and joint pain isn't very enjoyable, especially if you don't have any answers. But with good communication, any difficulties will be overshadowed by the feeling of closeness resulting from shared feelings and concerns.

The majority of this book has been directed toward the person with osteoarthritis. This chapter, however, has been designed for the non-OA person. This information can help you to see your loved one's unique experiences through his or her own eyes.

On to the Future

Well, you've just about finished this book. We've covered a lot of information about osteoarthritis. However, it's nice to know that research continues to investigate ways of improving the effectiveness of treatment.

Tremendous progress has been made in treatment for OA. Earlier diagnosis has led to earlier, more effective treatment, resulting in a better prognosis. Ongoing research continues to investigate the ways that joints function, as well as techniques that may decrease damage to bones and tissues and improve bone growth and repair. Finally, more attention is being given to find ways to further improve the quality of life for the person with OA.

Perhaps by the time you read this, some drug or treatment may have proven itself to be more successful than ones currently available. For example, recent research has been experimenting with drugs that may arrest cartilage degeneration. It remains to be seen whether these or other substances will improve your life with OA. But at least people are working on the problem.

It will take time to determine how effective these procedures and others will be in the treatment of OA. In addition, it is hoped that scientists may soon discover other types of treatments that may entirely eliminate osteoarthritis as a medical problem. Until then, hopefully you've learned a lot about how to cope with OA. Although it was impossible to include every possible problem that might be caused by OA in this text, I hope that what you've read will help you to develop your own strategies for coping.

Because things change, and something that troubles you one day may not trouble you the next (and vice versa), use this book as a resource. Whenever you have questions about how to cope with a certain aspect of osteoarthritis, consult these pages. If you have any comments—information you feel is important—or additional questions, feel free to write to me in care of the publisher. I'd be happy to hear from you. But for now, look brightly ahead, act proudly, and enjoy life as best you can. I wish all of my readers the very best of health and happiness!

Appendix

For further reading:

Lazarus, A. *In the Mind's Eye*. New York: Rawson Associates, 1977.

Linchitz, R. *Life Without Pain*. Reading, MA: Addison-Wesley Publishing Co., Inc., 1988.

For further information, contact:

Arthritis Foundation (National Office)
1314 Spring Street, N.W.
Atlanta, GA 30309

(404) 872-7100

National Chronic Pain Outreach
4922 Hampden Lane
Bethesda, MD 20814

(301) 652-4948

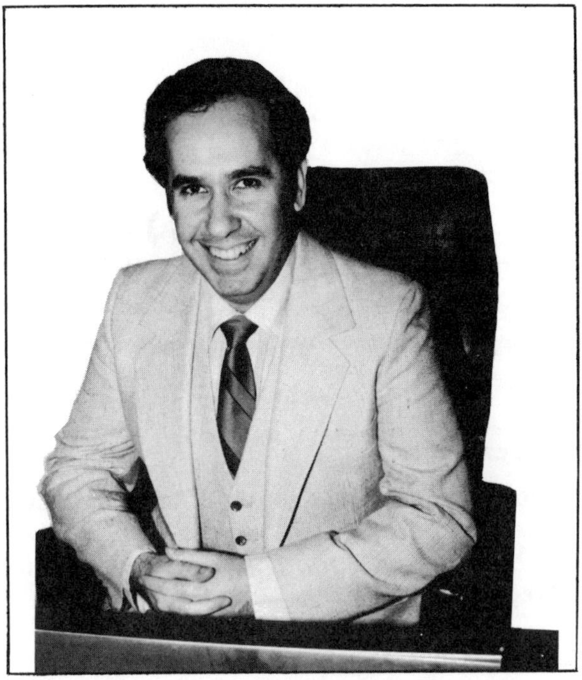

About the Author

Robert H. Phillips, Ph.D., is a practicing psychologist on Long Island, New York. He is the founder and director of the Center for Coping with Chronic Conditions, a multi-service organization helping individuals with chronic illness, and their families. He is involved with a number of local and national medical organizations. In addition, he is the psychologist for and director of the "Cope" program for the Long Island chapter of the Lupus Foundation of America, and is the associate director of the International Coma Recovery Institute.

The author of numerous articles on a variety of subjects in psychology, Dr. Phillips has lectured at conventions, universities, and professional meetings throughout the country, and has appeared on local and national radio and television programs.

Index